PRAISE FOR *THE PROVIDER COOKBOOK*

"An amazing book showcasing the best lifestyle! No one knows a connection to food better than a hunter. This book really showcases the bond between the tradition of hunting and the act of sharing an amazing meal with friends and family. It bridges the gap between food and the hunter's unique connection to the outdoors."

—REMI WARREN, *hunter, outdoor writer, and media personality*

"Ready to eat like royalty? You'll find so many new favorites in *The Provider Cookbook*, you'll wonder how you were preparing wild game and domestic meats without it. This is the rare book that truly feeds body, mind, and soul."

—GEORGE BRETT, *MLB Hall of Fame baseball player for the Kansas City Royals*

"Nothing is more rewarding than the feeling of preparing a meal literally from start to finish, with no 'middle men.' We as providers have full ability to ethically hunt, farm, and cook our own food, and it seems too many people are forgetting this—kudos to Belding and Mendes for keeping tradition alive."

—RILEY GREEN, *country music superstar*

"I've always loved the outdoors and sharing meals with family. This is so much more than just a cookbook!"

—MAX THIERIOT, *actor*

"Cooking is an art form, and Chad Belding and Chad Mendes understand that to their bones. Their passion shines through on every page of *The Provider Cookbook*."

—CHAD WARD, *founder of Whiskey Bent BBQ Supply*

"Feels almost weird to call this a cookbook because it's so much more . . . It's a tribute to a simpler time, to the 'call of the wild,' and to amazing dishes that nourish not only our bodies, but the long-starved human spirit."

—CLAY GUIDA, *fighter in the UFC Hall of Fame*

"Filled with stunning photos and mouth-watering recipes, *The Provider Cookbook* is truly something to savor. The stories within will inspire everyone who appreciates traditional methods of acquiring and preparing food."

—CODY "NO LOVE" GARBRANDT, *former MMA Bantamweight Champion*

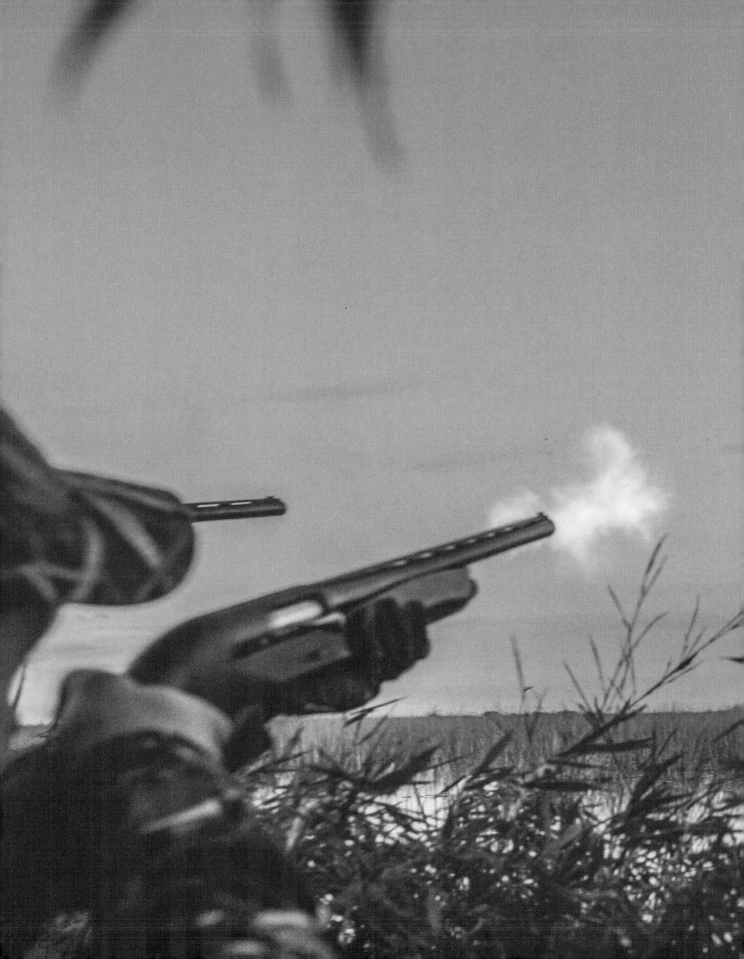

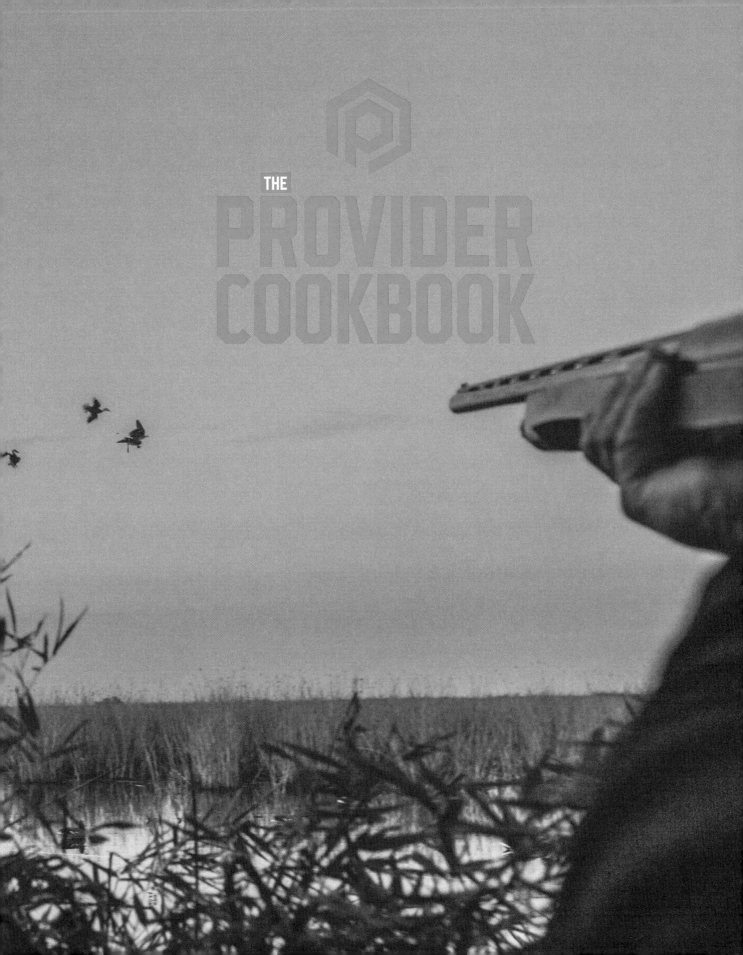

THE PROVIDER COOKBOOK

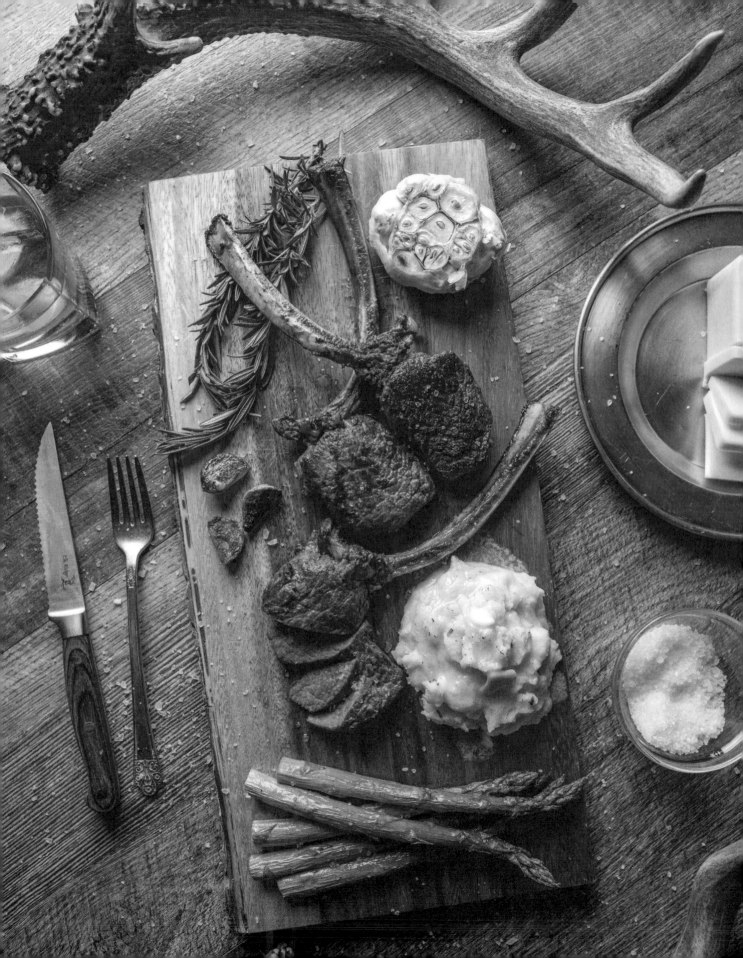

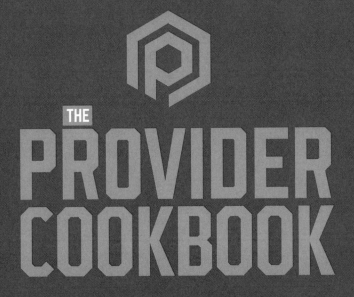

THE PROVIDER COOKBOOK

FISH AND GAME RECIPES FOR EATING WILD AND LIVING OFF THE LAND

CHAD BELDING AND CHAD MENDES

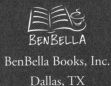

BENBELLA
BenBella Books, Inc.
Dallas, TX

3, 11, 74, and 93 by Keith Ailes, Muddy Shutter Media; pages 5, 6, 79, 215, 240–241, and 244 by Drew Seals, Nomad Collective; and page 51, courtesy of Chad Mendes. The following logos are pictured with permission: Banded; Finz & Feathers; Hunter Glenn Estate; Jack Daniel's; Kuiu; Lethal Products; MTN OPS; Napa Valley Olive Oil Mfg.; The Oyster Bed, LLC; Pelican Products, Inc.; The Provider, Realtree (courtesy of Jordan Outdoor Enterprises, Ltd.); Traeger Grills, LLC; and Vortex Optics.

BENBELLA

BenBella Books, Inc.
10440 N. Central Expressway, Suite 800
Dallas, TX 75231
benbellabooks.com
Send feedback to feedback@benbellabooks.com.

BenBella is a federally registered trademark.

Printed in the United States of America
10 9 8 7 6 5 4 3 2

Library of Congress Control Number: 2021020399
ISBN 978-1-637740-16-3
eISBN 978-1-637740-22-4

Editing by Claire Schulz
Copyediting by Karen Wise
Proofreading by Lisa Story and Amy Zarkos
Indexing by WordCo Indexing Services, Inc.
Text design by Aaron Edmiston
Cover design by Brigid Pearson
Printed by Versa Press

Special discounts for bulk sales are available.
Please contact bulkorders@benbellabooks.com.

To all of our friends, family, fellow hunters, and
Providers, this cookbook is dedicated to all of you!
Thank you for all the inspiration and passion.

CONTENTS

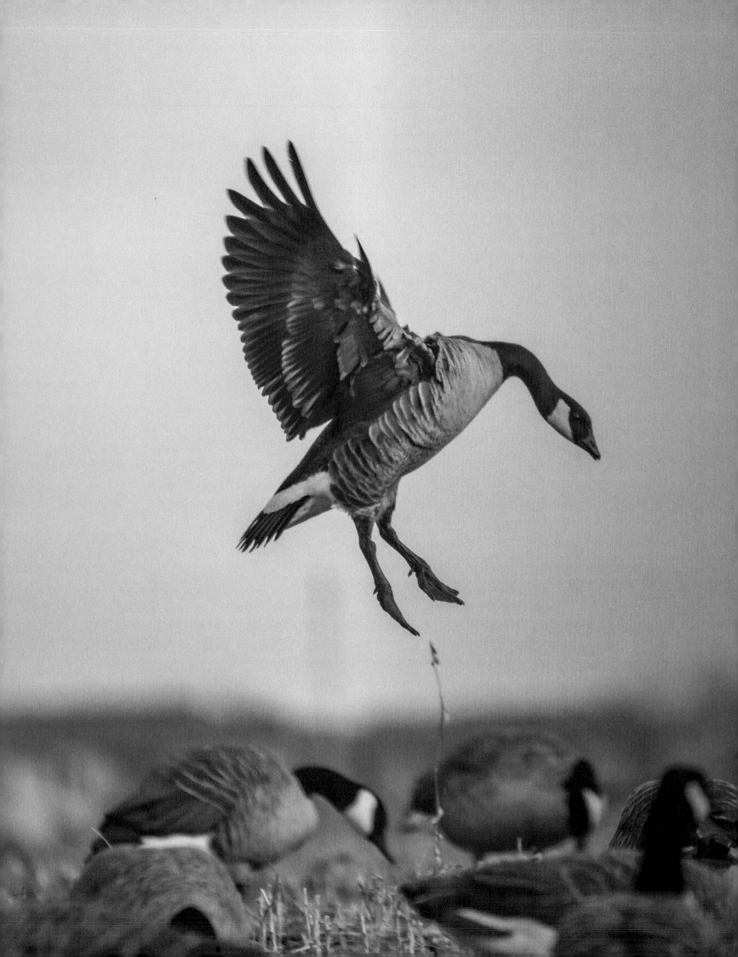

INTRODUCTION

Welcome, Provider! Pour yourself a cocktail and pull up a chair. With this cookbook, we're inviting you to our table to share in the amazing food and stories that we've accumulated from our travels hunting, fishing, and living off the land throughout the country.

WHO WE ARE

We are Chad Belding and Chad Mendes, both lifelong sportsmen and outdoor enthusiasts.

Chad Belding's love of this lifestyle was instilled from a very young age by his father, Orville Belding. Orville ensured that Chad and his brothers, Clay and Clint, developed appreciation of the outdoors, teaching them to camp, hunt, fish, trap crawdad, and even cut down their own Christmas trees. Their mother, Faith Belding, was with the family every step of the way. Chad's passion eventually led him to predator and waterfowl hunting, and soon thereafter he became involved in competitive duck and goose calling while attending college at the University of Nevada–Reno in the late 1990s. In school he was a member of the competitive Division I baseball team and studied business, public speaking, and history.

Following his graduation he put his business knowledge to good use, co-owning and operating several businesses across Nevada, Colorado, and Washington.

The call of the wilderness never left him, however, and in 2008 he founded Banded, a video production and merchandising company that specializes in hunting gear and accessories as well as duck and goose calls. The following year his TV show, *The Fowl Life*, aired, and the series has gotten more popular each year.

Chad Mendes was born and raised in Hanford, California. He still remembers following his dad through the Sierra Nevadas at six years old, staying at the family's go-to spots for fishing, and chasing blacktail and mule deer every season. At 13, he was lucky enough to kill his first buck in that mountain range, shooting an old PSE Nova bow that he had saved up for by mowing lawns. Hunting always had a special place in his heart, but it wasn't always his professional career. He had also grown up a talented wrestler. His success on the mat earned him a scholarship to California Polytechnic State University in San Luis Obispo, where his small-town palate opened up to a whole new world of cuisines. At Cal Poly he became a two-time Division I All-American wrestler. As a senior, he finished the year with a 30–1 record, placed second in the 2008 NCAA championships, and was named Pac-10 Wrestler of the Year. After graduating with a degree in kinesiology, he was invited to join Team Alpha Male, one of the best mixed martial arts (MMA) teams in the world. He quickly became a force on the regional mixed martial arts circuit and was signed with the Ultimate Fighting Championship in 2009. He competed for the UFC title three times against opponents like Conor McGregor and José Aldo.

Like Belding, Chad Mendes had a love of the outdoors that never left him. After retiring from the UFC, his experience and knowledge as a lifelong outdoorsman led him to create Finz and Featherz, a celebrity hunting and fishing service, which has grown into a successful business; and he became a brand ambassador for some prominent outdoor brands, including Traeger grills . . . which is how we first met.

As we hung out at Traeger events, then went on hunts and spent time together at hunting camps, we found out we had a lot in common—besides the fact that we're both named Chad! We were both college athletes. More than that, we both live for the outdoors and meeting people who share our passions for hunting, fishing, and cooking all sorts of wild game.

We have always felt a deep connection to our food and where it comes from. Belding followed in the footsteps of his dad and grandfather before him, who taught him the importance of living off the land and the pride of seeing your friends and family enjoy the bounty of the hunt. For Mendes, his love of food came from his family and also ties in with his wrestling career and focus on healthy eating for cutting weight. So we've both been cooking forever.

On *The Fowl Life*, Belding would cook up amazing dishes at duck camp, and viewers constantly told him, "I need that recipe!" The idea

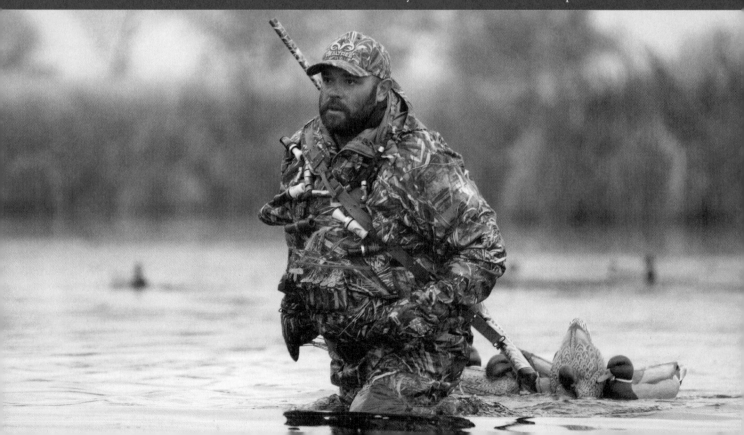

for a cookbook took hold, but he always felt he was too busy to sit down and write it. Meanwhile, Mendes would film his hunts and share them on YouTube, and viewers would watch him break down the animals and use them in great recipes. The more we talked about cooking and recipes, about traditions, and about what ethical hunting and fishing mean to us, we decided we had to bring the world our ideas of what it means to truly be a Provider.

BECOMING A PROVIDER

Hunting, fishing, and ethical farming have been a huge part of our lives, and we want to share these traditions. We want to pass them down from generation to generation and keep this lifestyle alive. To us, being a Provider is all about honing your skills as an ethical hunter, fisher, and gatherer, respecting and preserving animals and nature, keeping tradition alive, and bringing it all full circle by providing great meals for your friends and family.

BEING AN ETHICAL HUNTER AND FISHER

As hunters, fishers, gardeners, or farmers, we are privileged to know exactly where our food comes from. We sometimes forget that, though, because we're frequently around a lot of people of the same "thread count," if you will, who also see this lifestyle as second nature. But when we travel to many parts of the country, it's amazing to us how many people have never been introduced to a bow and arrow or a gun. So many people don't have that skill set that every hunter has.

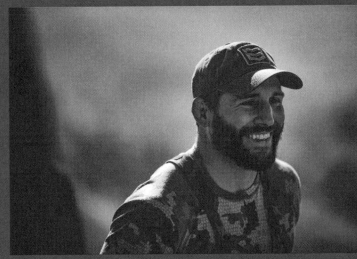

And yes, bringing down a duck or reeling in that fish—it's a rush. But it's not about the trophy. Compassion for the animal comes first. Always keep in mind that you are taking an animal's life for a reason—to put food on the table for your loved ones, and to do it in a way that preserves the animal's dignity.

RESPECTING AND PROTECTING MOTHER NATURE

Being a Provider also comes with a responsibility to respect the resource, learning how to protect our public and private lands where wildlife thrives. Hunters are the ultimate conservationists. As hunters and fishers, we understand that we are taking some animals out of the ecosystem, and we must ensure that wildlife populations and their habitats remain for many more generations to enjoy.

Hunters and outdoorsmen are also part of some of the biggest conservation efforts out there. From large organizations like Safari Club International, Mule Deer Foundation, and Pheasants Forever to local agencies like the California Waterfowl Association, they have invested a lot of sweat equity in protecting animals and their habitat as precious natural resources. For instance, the National Wild Turkey Federation, which stands behind conservation and hunters' rights, brought the wild turkey back from the brink of extinction. They continue to work to put more turkeys in the fields. The Rocky Mountain Elk Foundation has done an incredible job of putting more Rocky Mountain elk, tule elk, and Roosevelt elk back into the mountains through predator control and feeding programs. They take sleds of hay into areas so that elk can still have a healthy diet on their breeding grounds. The California Waterfowl Association has done amazing wetlands work to protect duck habitat—not just where ducks feed but where they nest, keeping those eggs safe from predators. Communication with and education of farmers is also a part of this—for instance, with their egg salvage program. Twenty or thirty years ago, if a farmer saw a duck hen fly off her nest, he would probably keep right on clearing the field, and his equipment would tear up that nest and all those duck eggs. Now,

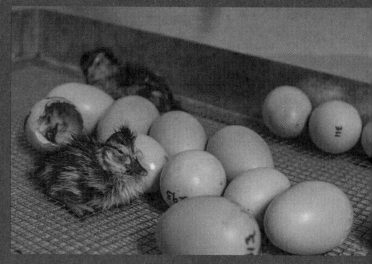

organizations work with farmers to send biologists onto farmland to pick up that nest, bring the eggs to an incubation site to hatch, and return those ducks to wild marshes. They save thousands of eggs every year. Chad Belding's uncle Mel is part of an agency called Nevada Bighorns Unlimited, which has a program to install guzzlers on mountain ranges. These guzzlers collect rainwater for wildlife to access during dry periods when a drought might kill them. But it's not just the bighorn sheep that benefit; wild horses, sage hens, chukars, and coyotes in these areas also take advantage of the guzzlers.

All of this is made possible through the sale of yearly hunting and trapping licenses and tags. The revenue from US license sales is more than $1 billion every year, and by law that license money goes directly to state wildlife and conservation programs.

Hunters also donate money and volunteer their time to support these projects—working the banquets and raising money through silent auctions and raffles to protect habitat. The two of us not only spend a lot of money on conservation initiatives but also volunteer our time

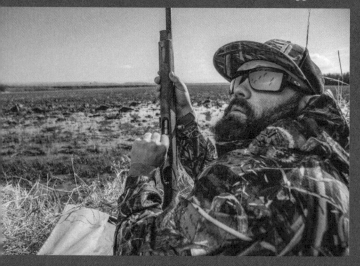

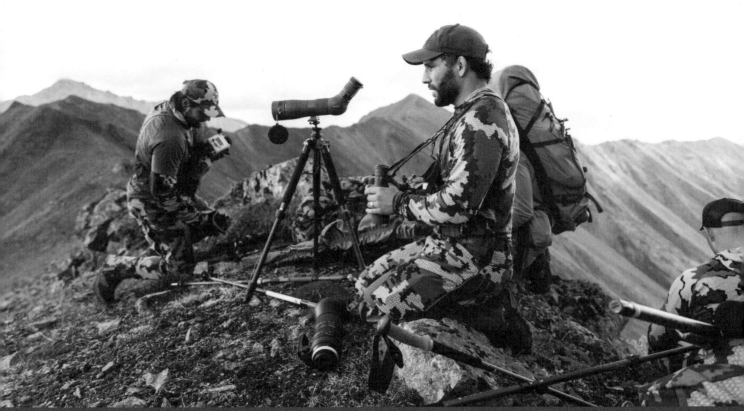

to support conservation agencies that protect wildlife of all types against disease, population overgrowth, and industrial and residential spread. We see this as part of our responsibility as Providers.

Today's hunters are also taking some pretty cool steps to manage populations on their property. Say you own 200 acres and there's a white-tail deer population on your land. Land owners can set up trail cameras that snap a photo when an animal walks by. This can give you an amazingly accurate inventory of those deer—their maturity level, their numbers, what kinds of deer are on your property at what times of year. This then allows you to pick and choose. If you see a healthy buck that's only three years old, you can decide to let him grow for another few years to reproduce and instead harvest only a certain age class. So now you have a healthy herd that's not overpopulated or overhunted.

We don't know who could do this work without hunters. Many of the environmental and animal rights organizations out there are anti-hunting. We don't want to fight with these groups—we share a goal with them of protecting animals and habitat. So we just want to educate them on everything hunters and fishers are doing in this space. Hunters are the ones who are reacting to the problems and taking the necessary actions to get it done. For sure, hunters are conservationists first and foremost.

KEEPING TRADITION ALIVE

Being a Provider also means becoming a mentor and introducing new men, women, and kids to the outdoors and the culture of the American hunter. As we said, we sometimes take it for granted that everybody knows about this lifestyle, but they don't. In recent years, hunting has become less popular nationally. For instance, there were 13.6 million hunters in America in 2011, and that number dropped

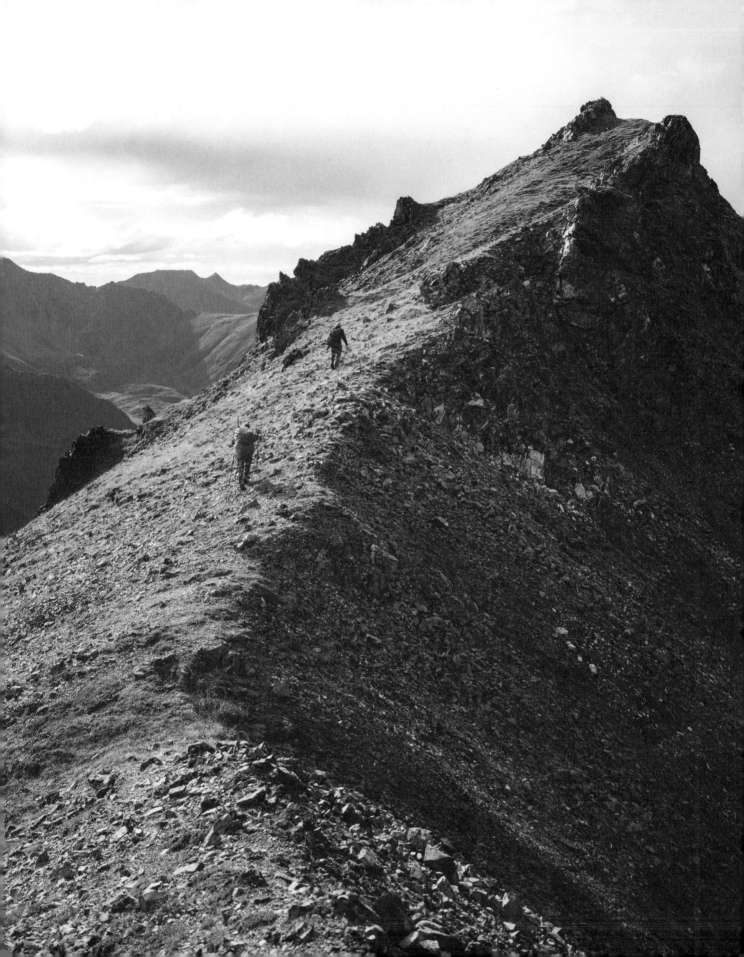

to 11.4 million in 2016. That's a problem for those conservation agencies that depend on the fees hunters pay for licenses.

We do see signs that hunting and fishing are due for a revival. During COVID-19, hunting license sales surged, including for hunters between the ages of 10 and 16. The two of us got so many new people asking us, "How do I get a gun? How do I go turkey hunting?" Chad Mendes's company has seen many brand-new hunters—both men and women—in recent years. We also work with college kids at UC Davis, which offers a new hunter program to juniors and seniors, and has a 70 percent return rate of new hunters to the field. The fastest-growing demographic in hunting is women. If you look at the industry today, you'll see new clothing, bows, guns, all of it specialized for women. All of this is encouraging.

And all it takes is the right mentoring program. We've seen it happen so many times. We bring someone new to camp, teach them gun safety, how to pluck a duck, cook that duck into something delicious . . . they get utterly taken up with it and want to come back again. We firmly believe that if we open our eyes to the idea of teaching somebody new—even one person a season—we're going to keep this tradition alive for generations to come.

HEALTH AND THE HUNT

For us, the health benefits of wild game greatly outweigh the benefits of store-bought domestic meat. When you harvest wild game, as we've said, you know exactly where that meat came from. As an ethical hunter, you know that that animal lived well and was killed humanely. During its life, it was not raised on feed laced with antibiotics or GMOs.

Chad Mendes will tell you that during his wrestling career and UFC training camps, he felt so much better when he'd eat wild game compared to eating conventional domestic meat. He'd be putting his body through incredible stress, doing two- and three-hour workouts. If he ate domestic beef, he would notice even

A Word on Predator Control

As Providers, we truly value hunting and fishing to bring in food for our families. But there's another side to hunting, and that's predator control. We have to respect all animals. We don't disrespect a coyote just because we wouldn't eat a coyote or because it has a reputation as a predator. We have to understand that we have built our homes and communities on their land, and they're fighting for that same space.

At the same time, if we don't keep predators in check, they can also threaten wildlife populations. Foxes kill a million adult ducks a year (and that's on top of the eggs they also eat). So we as hunters also have a responsibility to manage the predator population.

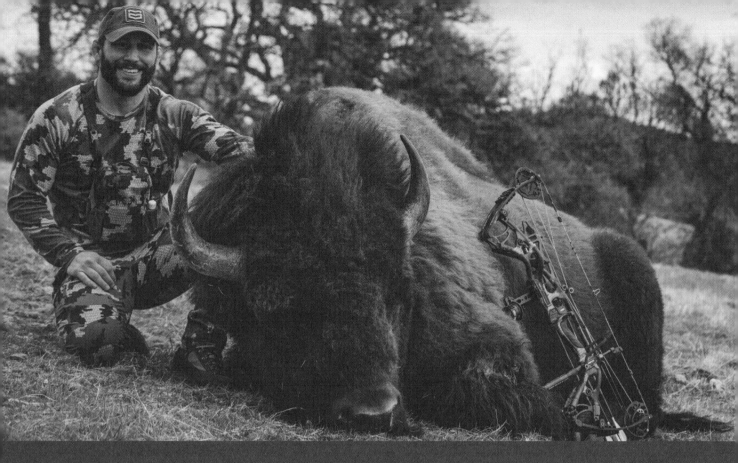

going into practice that he felt tired and sluggish and just didn't have much enthusiasm. But he felt much better when he was eating wild game.

Part of that is because wild game is very lean, especially when you compare it to something like Wagyu beef, which is much higher in fat. Obviously you can still get great effects from a diet of healthy store-bought meat (and we still enjoy beef, pork, and chicken—we even include recipes for those in this book!). For Mendes, what was more important was that hunting allowed him to recharge. Doing all of the media interviews, working to cut weight, going through a fight camp, and then competing in front of so many people—it all created a huge disconnect. Afterward, he needed to get away for a bit, so he'd take a week and hike into the backcountry to chase elk. It was a way for him to recharge his soul and get his mindset back to where he needed

to be. Bringing your skills to provide for yourself and your family strengthens you and makes you feel better mentally and emotionally. (Not to mention, hunters and fishers need to be in good form to pursue animals! To that end, Mendes shares some of his top training tips on page 190.)

After hunting, Mendes was refreshed and could carry that feeling of accomplishment back with him. Being a Provider recharges your battery and helps you get ready to return to the rest of your life with more energy and enthusiasm. Now, hunting might never be how you get all your protein. You might be able to bring down only five ducks a year. But with the pride of being a Provider, you're going to put every bit of your passion and love into preparing those five ducks for your loved ones. So for us, the health benefits of this lifestyle are more about the mentality and how it strengthens your soul.

SHARING THE LOVE

The connection that Providers have with our food is something we always cherish. You get out there, make a kill, have a harvest, and now you have all this incredible high-quality meat that will feed many of your friends and family. Harvesting a deer, for example, will get you 50 to 70 pounds of fresh, free-range meat.

We love to be in nature and the experiences that come with being in the field, the camaraderie we share with the people at our camp. It all comes full circle when you take that game, fish, or fowl you brought in and turn it into amazing meals. For the two of us, cooking is just as rewarding as the hunt itself. Even when we're out in the field, we're already picturing what that meal might be like—the spices we'll put into it, the accompaniments we'll serve on the side.

There just is no better feeling than sharing this food with people and hearing, "Oh my gosh, is that really wild duck?" or, "I've never had venison taste like this before!" We love to share our bounty with friends—they get so creative with it. Maybe you're interested in cooking with game but aren't a hunter yet. We think that's awesome. If you want to try game, you may be able to purchase farm-raised deer, elk, or boar. But in our view that will never compete with having a hunter share a tenderloin along with the story of where it came from. So make friends with a hunter . . . or try to hunt yourself!

IN THIS BOOK

This is a celebration of the Provider life, with recipes and stories from memorable hunts. We'll take you on a journey into hunting camps (and backyard barbecues) where we have enjoyed great food and great conversations with other Providers.

In this cookbook, we include not just our own recipes but dishes that our friends

Field and Farm to Fork

It's so important to know where your food comes from and how it was treated before it ended up on your plate. A lot of beef, pork, and chicken is inhumanely raised. That's coming to light more and more, which we think is part of why hunting is maintaining its traction and may appeal to a whole new wave of outdoorsmen and women. Thankfully, these days many more food companies are being transparent about the way they raise their animals, telling the story of how their cattle, pigs, or chickens are treated. People want it done ethically and correctly. We like to support many smaller mom-and-pop type farms that offer free-range meat and eggs. Before you buy, do your research. Go online first, check out the brands, and see what's going on. A Provider knows where their food came from and can feel good about sharing it with their family.

and family have shared with us. We want to highlight the camaraderie and connection that are inherent parts of the hunting and fishing lifestyle. People who hunt and fish share a passion for the outdoors and a love of food. It just comes with being at hunting camp or cooking in the kitchen or over an open fire. When you meet someone else who hunts, you hear their field stories and you start talking about all the recipes you've made with different types of wild game. It inspires you to try their foods and maybe even put your own spin on it. We're celebrating our fellow hunters and fishers who have influenced us over the years and made us better chefs.

These recipes have broadened our view of just how creative one can be with big game like deer and wild boar, upland game birds such as pheasants and quail, waterfowl, and all the fish we can catch. You'll find everything from classic comfort foods and tasty sandwiches and tacos on up to more involved dishes like Antelope Backstrap Roulade and Pan-Seared Specklebelly Goose with Port Wine–Cherry Reduction. We also share a chapter of our favorite recipes for domestic beef, pork, and chicken. If you're wondering what to serve alongside these meals, check out the last chapter, which has amazing sides and sauces.

In many recipes you'll see that we recommend specific brands of ingredients and equipment. Of course, you can still get great results if you use whatever you have on hand. But we invite you to try the offerings from these companies if you can. Here's a bit more about them:

Traeger is a manufacturer of wood-fired pellet grills. As we mentioned, we've worked with them for years now, and we think their offerings are next-level. The flavor that grilling with wood pellets creates is unbelievable, but

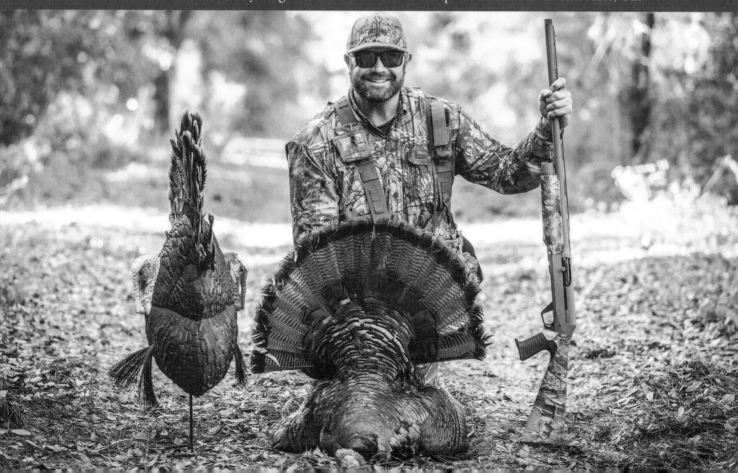

the ease of use is the biggest thing. Rather than messing around with charcoal and lighter fluid, you turn a dial, the grill ignites, and it holds that temperature. Anybody can become a pit master! And many of the people who work at the company are invested in the outdoors and living off the land; we know that they value the Provider way of life. That said, you can of course make these recipes with a gas or charcoal grill and the dishes will still taste good—it's a matter of preference and what you have available. But if you have the means, we highly recommend Traeger.

The Oyster Bed is a small military member–owned company that offers a wonderful line of grill- and oven-safe cookware. Oyster Beds are made from a lightweight metal alloy that can withstand temperatures up to a thousand degrees. They're molded with small reservoirs that hold the juices from whatever you're cooking. Hailing from Louisiana, the founders, brothers Tommy and Adam Waller, deeply understand how important oysters are to the world's marine ecosystems. They donate a portion of their proceeds back to ocean research and conservation. (We don't have a formal relationship with this company—we just love their product and their mission!) Oyster Beds are available at select spots throughout the US and online. If you don't have one yet, we recommend using a cast-iron skillet instead.

We've also included a few recipes for *Jack Daniel's* cocktails. We're sure you've heard of Jack Daniel's whiskey! We appreciate their support for conservation efforts through ad

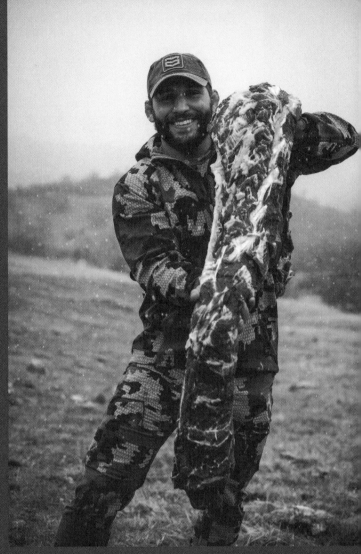

campaigns and habitat investment over the years. (Plus, there's nothing like sipping on a great craft cocktail while you cook!)

We hope these recipes and stories will satisfy your appetite and inspire you to connect more deeply with your food and where it comes from.

The Provider Rubs

Several of these recipes feature our signature spice rubs, which are absolutely amazing on wild game and fish and also great on domestic meats and sides. You can get yours online at www.theproviderlife.com.

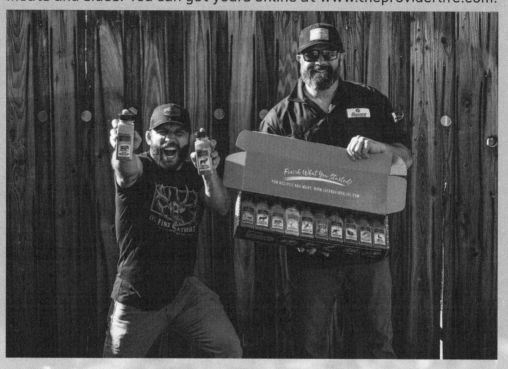

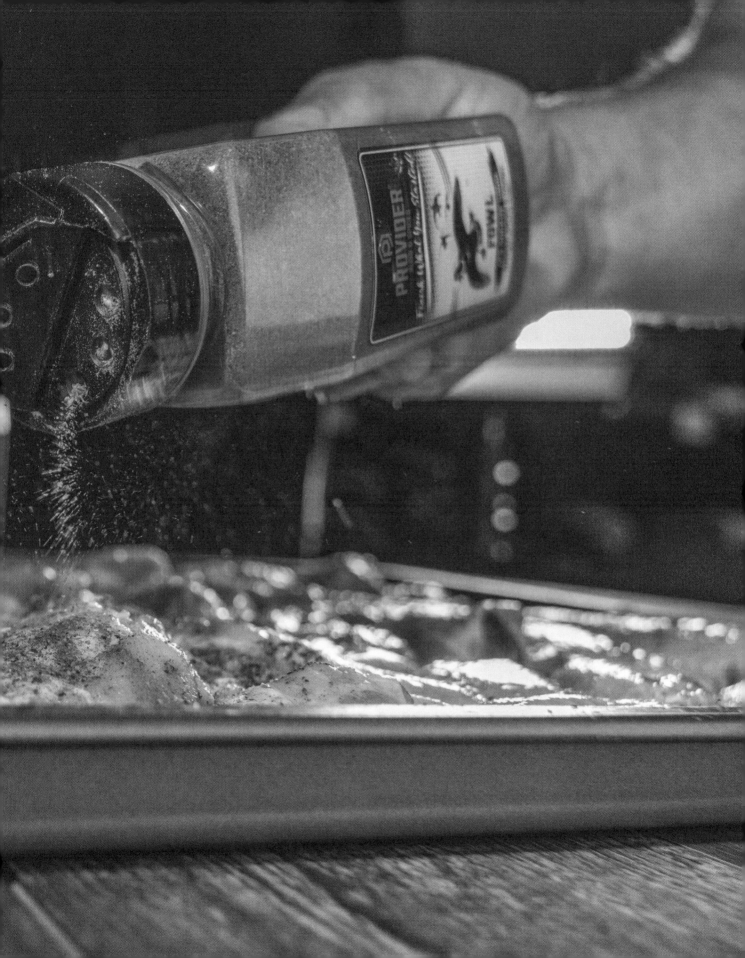

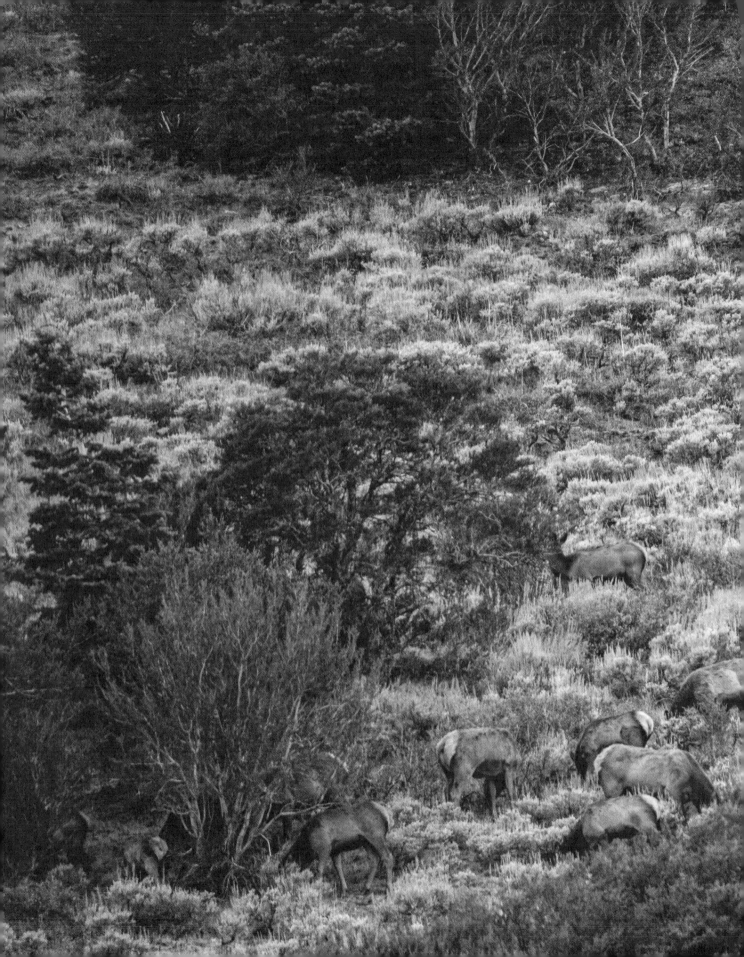

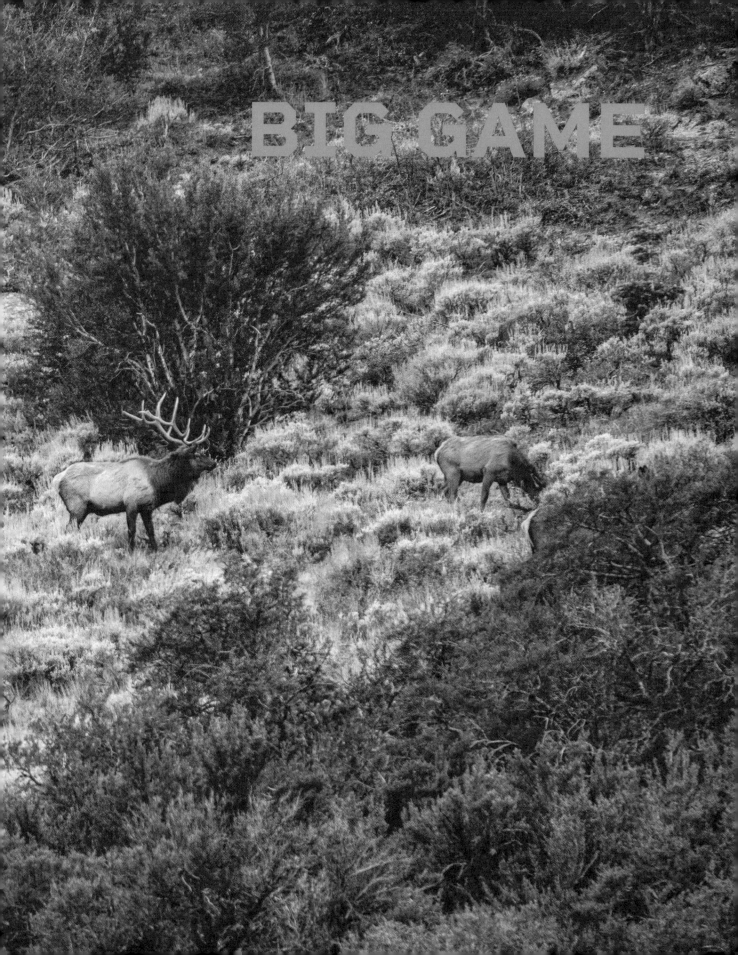

BIG GAME

Venison tenderloins and backstraps are a real treat, and a big set of velvet-covered antlers makes a great decoration for the table! During a banner year for water in the Nevada desert, Chad Belding's brothers, Clint and Clay, and their friend Alex had archery mule deer tags in their pockets and visions of a group of big bucks they had spotted the year prior during an antelope hunt. But an early scouting trip had the guys reeling as they were unable to turn up the bucks they had spotted the year before. With each hunt the team learned more about this herd of Nevada mule deer, and with each hunt they knew it was not going to be easy to harvest *one* of these deer, let alone three of them.

As time ticked away toward opening day, the guys knew they had to make a decision: keep looking for this group, or move to a new location and start over. Not wanting to risk it all, they decided to stay put.

Clay would be the first in camp, arriving a day ahead of Clint and Alex. He had one solo day to scout before the opening morning hunts. As Clint and Alex steamed toward camp, their phones rang. "Do you want a 26-inch 9-by-7 or a 28-inch 4-by-4?" Clay calmly asked. He had found the bucks; now all that was left to do was . . . everything!

The night before opening day, nobody got any sleep as visions of perfectly placed arrows danced in their heads. The morning's

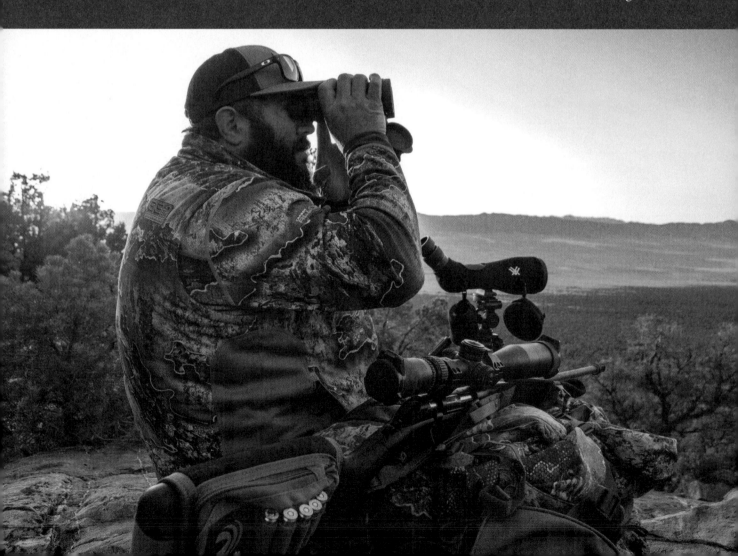

hunt brought a close encounter with the target bucks, but no arrows were flung. Archery hunting in August means a lot of downtime midday, a perfect time to build blinds, plan hunts, and shoot bows in the sweltering heat.

Glass, strategize, hunt, and repeat became the routine for the next few days. Any time spent in the outdoors is better than work, but frustration and dark thoughts of unfilled tags crept in. Four days into the hunt and none of the guys had even drawn their bows. This group of elusive bucks had seemingly different behaviors every day, and establishing a pattern was not going to happen. The guys were going to need a lot of luck in order to notch those tags.

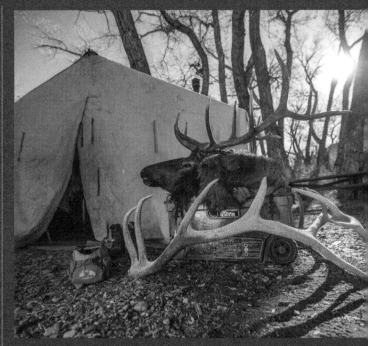

After five days of unsuccessful hunting, they were beginning to think they should have stayed home. However, the group of bucks had made a pass through a patch of tall sagebrush in the days prior, and judging by the patterns in the beat-down game trail, Clint and Alex had a feeling they might do it again. Clay had chosen a different area and was unable to close the distance on the bucks due to lack of cover. As they watched the sun go down, they feared the deer would not make it into bow range before shooting light was gone.

As the last minutes of the shooting light faded away, the deer suddenly made a beeline for the tall sagebrush where Alex and Clint lay in wait. The 26-inch nontypical buck busted up in front of Alex at 17 yards and turned broadside, and there was no need to look at him for long before he knew this buck was the one. A well-placed arrow and Alex had the largest deer of his life: 195 inches and some change. That dream buck had the guys on cloud nine all night, even knowing there was still work left to be done in the morning.

Clint unfortunately had to head home after night five's festivities, but Alex and Clay remained, questing for another buck. Morning six was just like the first five, close but no cigar. This was a crucial point in time for the hunt. Alex and Clay had one deer hanging in the Nevada heat that needed to get cooled off or back to town for processing, but they desperately wanted to fill Clay's tag. They decided to stay for the evening hunt, which meant breaking down Alex's deer in the field so it could be placed in a cooler. The guys spent the day butchering the recently harvested venison and even grilled up a little bit of the highly coveted tenderloins. Once this work was done, it was time to get back on the hunt.

Clay decided to hit the same sagebrush patch Alex and Clint had hunted the night before. The target deer began to roam around about an hour before sunset, a good and bad thing as the two watched them frolic around at 300 yards with no way to close any distance.

As the group of deer fed away from the sagebrush patch, Clay and Alex thought they were finished. Suddenly the 28-inch 4-by-4 broke away from the group and walked right to the patch of sagebrush—the stroke of luck Clay had needed all week long. The majestic buck stood alone, 7 yards in front of Clay, seeming somewhat of an offering after a long week's hunt. Clay's arrow found its mark perfectly, and he too now held the largest deer of his hunting career, just a shade over the ultimate goal of 200 inches. The trip was finally complete.

Hard work and determination paid off for the guys, and they were rewarded with freezers full of organic meat, trophies for the wall, and memories to last a lifetime. Sadly, Clint would not return to camp after having an old neck injury come back to haunt him, leaving him unable to draw a bow. He would, however, be rewarded for his hard work with a backstrap dinner prepared to perfection by Clay and Alex. Good friends, good hunts, and good meals—it doesn't get much better than that!

In this chapter, you'll find recipes for big game like deer, elk, and boar.

Sausage Grinding

Providing for our families is a constant grind. Long hours of work require the ability to prepare good, nutritious meals quickly. Wild game can serve as an important piece of the puzzle. Venison and fowl can provide high-protein, low-fat options for your family. Grinding your wild game is a great way to diversify meal options.

We like to add some pork fat to our game or dark fowl proteins. It greatly enhances the flavor and consistency. Pork shoulder (also known as pork butt) is a great choice to add to your grind. Contact your local butcher and have them prepare the shoulder with as little trimming as possible. We recommend the grind to be a ratio of 75/25 to 80/20 mixture of game to pork.

The sky is the limit when it comes to flavors. Some of our favorites are butt burger (no added spices), chorizo, and sweet and hot Italian sausage. Think of the pasta dishes, burgers, soups, or tacos that you can throw together quickly and easily while always providing for your friends and family!

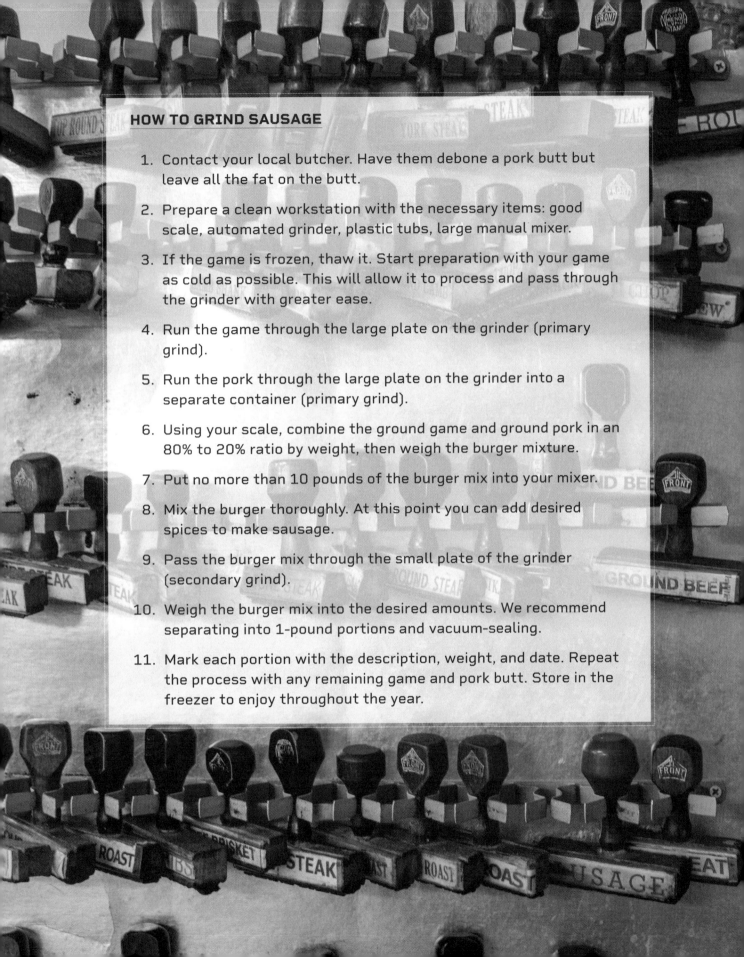

HOW TO GRIND SAUSAGE

1. Contact your local butcher. Have them debone a pork butt but leave all the fat on the butt.

2. Prepare a clean workstation with the necessary items: good scale, automated grinder, plastic tubs, large manual mixer.

3. If the game is frozen, thaw it. Start preparation with your game as cold as possible. This will allow it to process and pass through the grinder with greater ease.

4. Run the game through the large plate on the grinder (primary grind).

5. Run the pork through the large plate on the grinder into a separate container (primary grind).

6. Using your scale, combine the ground game and ground pork in an 80% to 20% ratio by weight, then weigh the burger mixture.

7. Put no more than 10 pounds of the burger mix into your mixer.

8. Mix the burger thoroughly. At this point you can add desired spices to make sausage.

9. Pass the burger mix through the small plate of the grinder (secondary grind).

10. Weigh the burger mix into the desired amounts. We recommend separating into 1-pound portions and vacuum-sealing.

11. Mark each portion with the description, weight, and date. Repeat the process with any remaining game and pork butt. Store in the freezer to enjoy throughout the year.

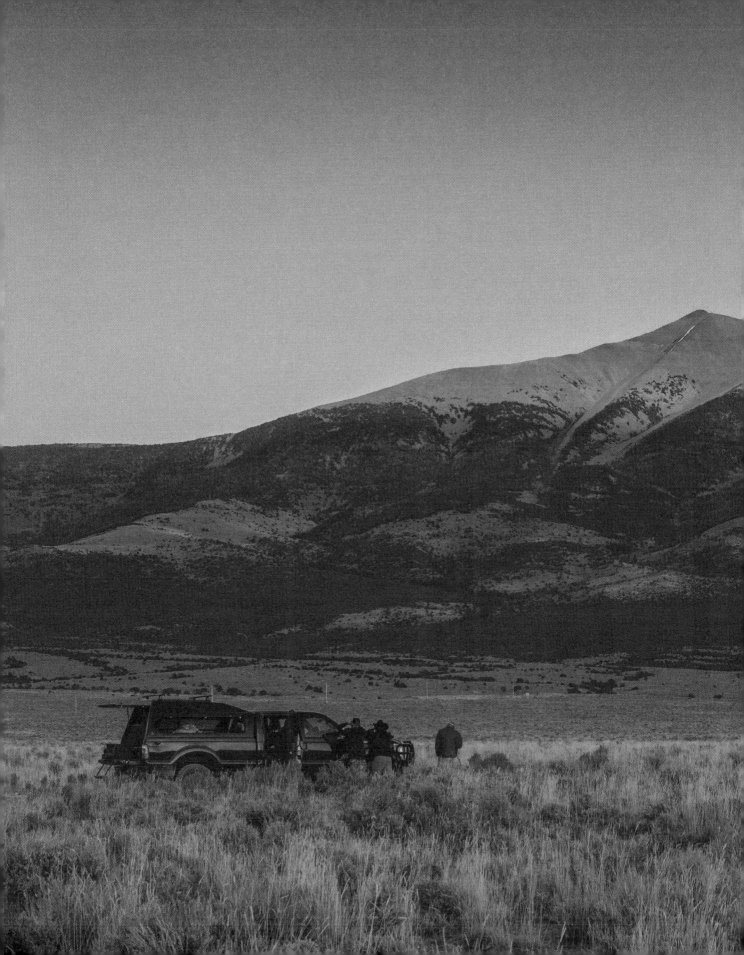

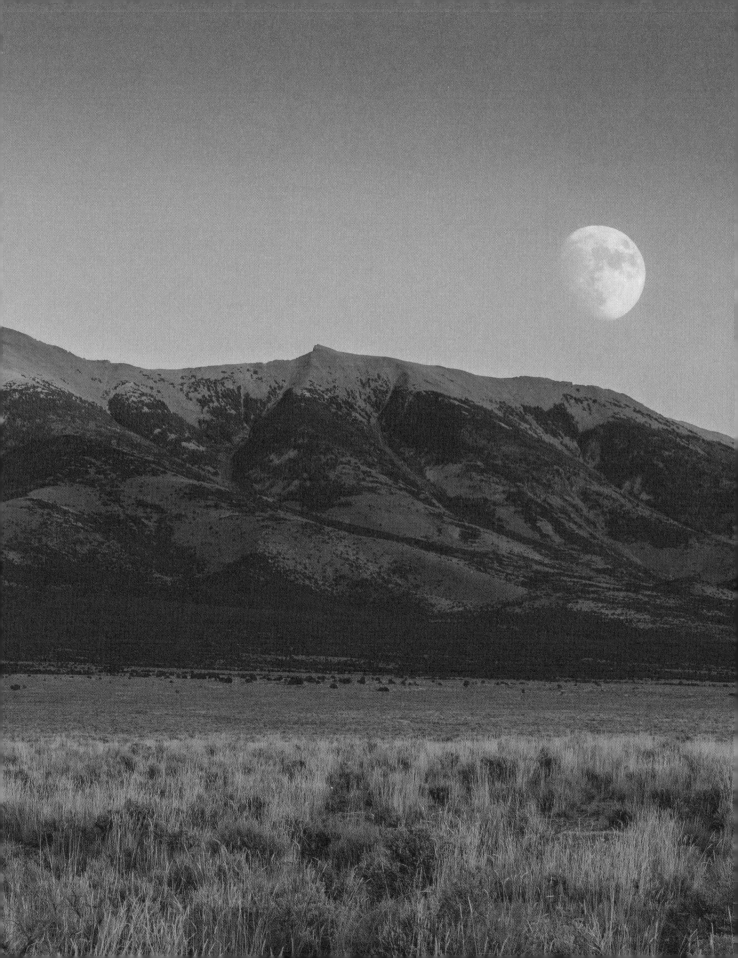

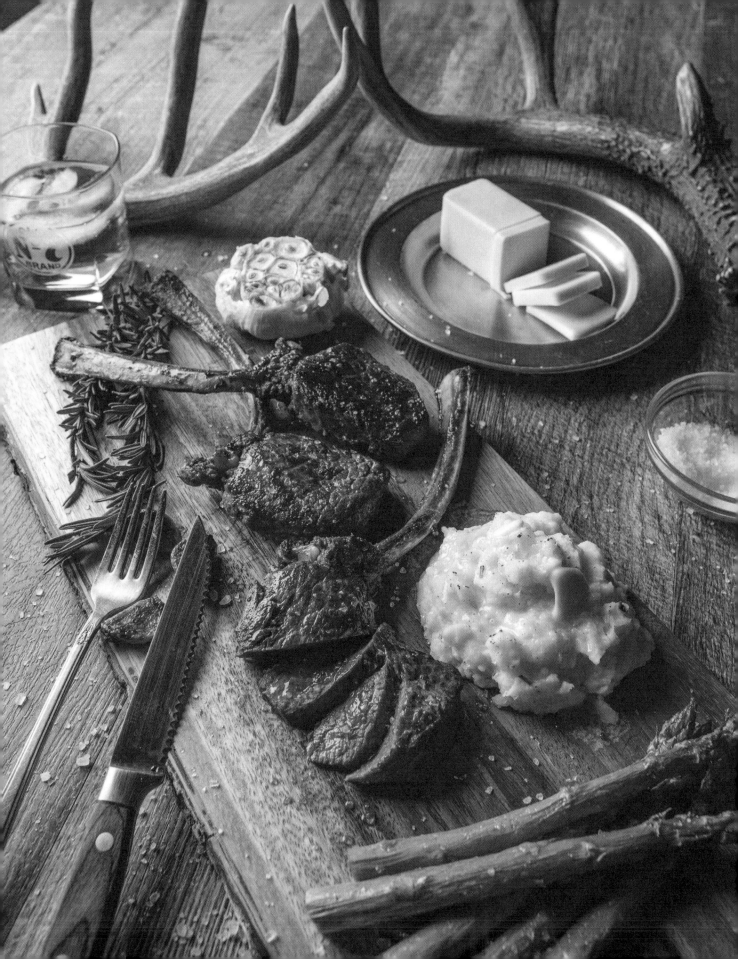

Smoked Venison Tomahawk Steaks

SERVES 4–6

The tomahawk is the part of the rib bone that's still attached to the backstrap, and any wild game tomahawk steaks can be used in this recipe. Adding smoke before searing in butter, garlic, and rosemary gives them amazing flavor. Make sure you don't overcook them. These pair really nicely with a full-bodied red wine!

4–6 venison tomahawk steaks (about 1 inch thick)

1–2 tablespoons salt

1–2 tablespoons ground black pepper

4 tablespoons (½ stick) unsalted butter

3–4 garlic cloves, peeled and lightly smashed

4–5 fresh rosemary sprigs

Season both sides of the steaks with the salt and pepper.

Set your grill/smoker (we use a Traeger) to 165°F and heat for 15 minutes. Place the steaks on the grate and smoke for about 1 hour, until the internal temperature hits 115°F.

Toward the end of the smoke time, place a cast-iron skillet over high heat on your stovetop. Melt the butter in the skillet. When the steaks are done smoking, transfer them directly to the skillet; the skillet should be hot enough that you hear a strong sizzle. Add the garlic cloves and rosemary sprigs. Scoop the melted butter, garlic, and rosemary around and on top of the steaks as they sear. Cook until they reach the desired temperature (135–140°F is medium-rare for venison), 2–3 minutes each side. Transfer the steaks to plates and enjoy immediately.

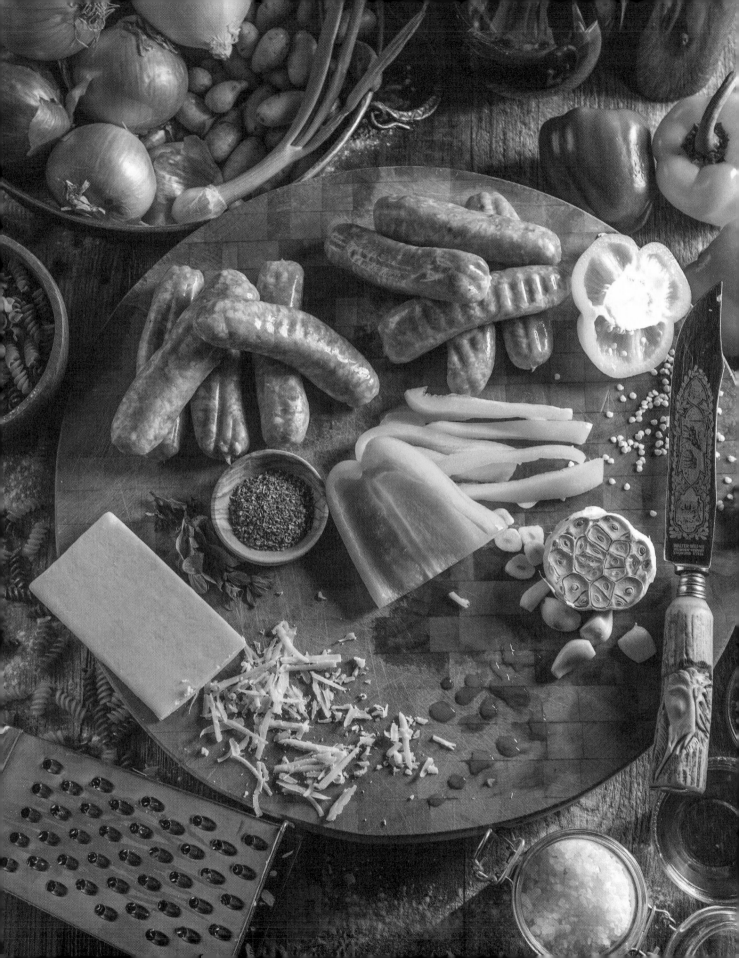

Fillipone Elk Sausage and Peppers

SERVES 4

This Italian-style sausage and pepper recipe has been passed down from generation to generation within the Fillipone family. It just so happens that Chad Belding's uncle Glenn Fillipone has mastered it, and that is why it has become a staple at all of our family and holiday gatherings! The flavors and ingredients are blended perfectly to keep your mouth watering with anticipation of every bite. Saluti and buon appetito!

---

10 ounces rainbow rotini

1 pound elk sausage, sliced

3 pounds sweet Italian pork sausage, sliced

1 cup half-and-half, divided

½ cup chopped fresh parsley

1 tablespoon dried crushed marjoram

½ teaspoon salt

⅛ teaspoon ground black pepper

1 cup chopped sweet yellow onion

5 garlic cloves, minced

3 bell peppers (one green, one red, one orange), seeded and chopped

2 tablespoons all-purpose flour

½ cup grated parmesan cheese, plus more for serving

Bring a large pot of water to a boil. Cook the rotini according to package directions. Drain well and set aside.

Heat a large frying pan over medium-high heat. Brown the elk sausage and Italian sausage.

While the sausage is cooking, in a large saucepan, bring ¾ cup of the half-and-half to a gentle simmer over medium-low heat. Add the parsley, marjoram, salt, and pepper.

When the sausage has browned, transfer to a plate lined with paper towels to drain. Pour off all but about 1 tablespoon of the drippings from the pan.

continued

Add the onion and garlic to the frying pan and cook until softened. Add the bell peppers and return the sausage to the pan.

In a small bowl, whisk the flour with the remaining ¼ cup half-and-half. Add it to the simmering sauce mixture, bring to a slow boil, and whisk until thickened.

Add the parmesan to the sauce, reduce the heat to medium, and cook just until the cheese melts. Remove the saucepan from the heat. Add the sausage and veggie mixture to the saucepan, along with the cooked pasta. Stir until blended and heated through and serve with additional parmesan for garnish.

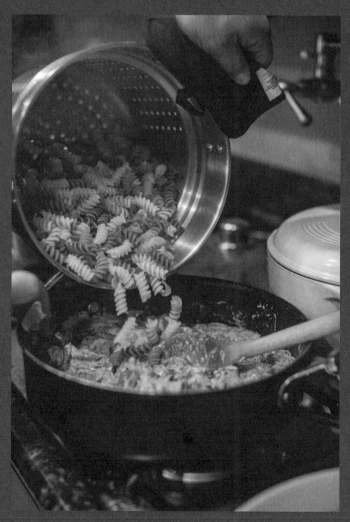
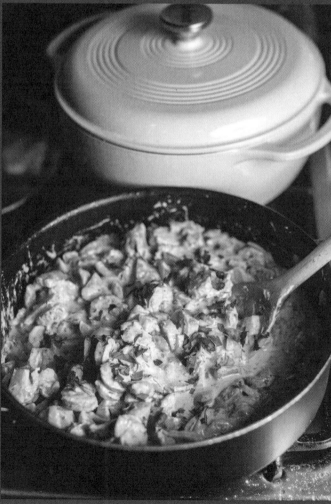

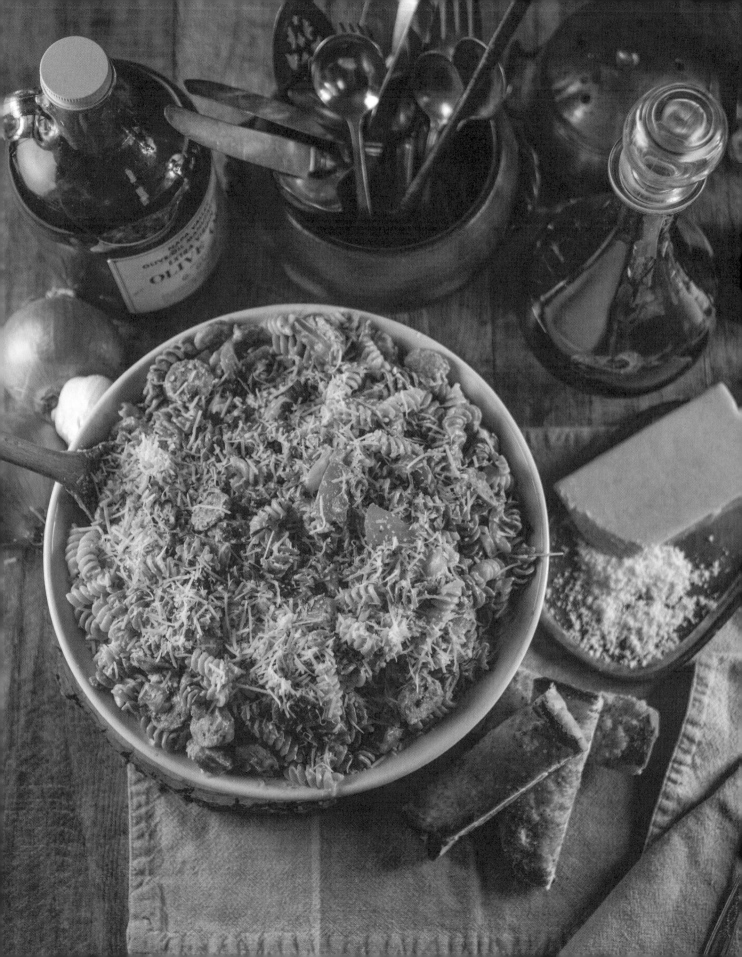

Mr. Billy's Smothered Deer Steaks

SERVES 6

As hunters we all have our niche. Turns out Chad Belding's is mallard ducks. But who knew through hunting ducks he would find his favorite deer recipe? As he tells it, "Hunting ducks led me straight to the mallard capital of the world: Arkansas. The historical flooded timbers made a duck hunter's paradise. Although it was the mallards that originally took me to the state, it was the people who kept me coming back. Among those remarkable people like Brandon, Joel, Todd, Chris, and many others, I stumbled upon the great Mr. Billy Bogey. His love for hunting and cooking would lead me to countless hours of conversation while making everything from wild game, frog legs, and fried bologna sandwiches to some of the best blackberry cobbler you've ever tried. The list goes on and on, but it would not be complete without Mr. Billy's famous smothered deer steaks. I have eaten deer well over 3,000 times. And not one of those 3,000 times could ever compare to the first time I ever tried this dish—I mean not even close. You could cut it with a freakin' fork. That gravy grabbed my attention in a hurry, and then the flavor of the meat brought me to my knees! (Thank God I could still reach for seconds from the floor.) This deer steak changed my life and I hope it has the same effect on you!"

---

2 pounds deer steaks (preferably from the hind quarter or shoulder), pounded flat

2 cups all-purpose flour

1 tablespoon Cajun seasoning (Mr. Billy likes Tony Chachere's)

1 tablespoon Greek seasoning

1 cup neutral vegetable oil

2 (12-ounce) jars brown gravy

1 red bell pepper, seeded and sliced thinly

1 green bell pepper, seeded and sliced thinly

1 white onion, thinly sliced

2 jalapeños, seeded and sliced (optional)

Preheat the oven to 250°F.

In a shallow dish, mix the flour with the Cajun seasoning and Greek seasoning. Dredge the steaks in the flour mixture to coat, then shake off the excess.

Heat the vegetable oil to 400°F in a large cast-iron skillet. Add the deer steaks and deep-fry for 2 minutes per side (they will be only halfway done).

While the steaks are frying, bring the gravy to a boil in a small saucepan over medium heat.

Transfer the half-done steaks to a Dutch oven or large, heavy-bottomed pot and add the bell peppers and onion. Pour the boiling-hot gravy over the deer meat. Add the jalapeños, if desired, and cover the pot with the lid or aluminum foil.

Transfer the pot to the oven and bake for 3 hours, until the gravy is at your desired thickness and you can cut the deer steaks with a fork.

Mr. Billy says: "Serve with mashed potatoes or rice. And don't forget the sweet tea."

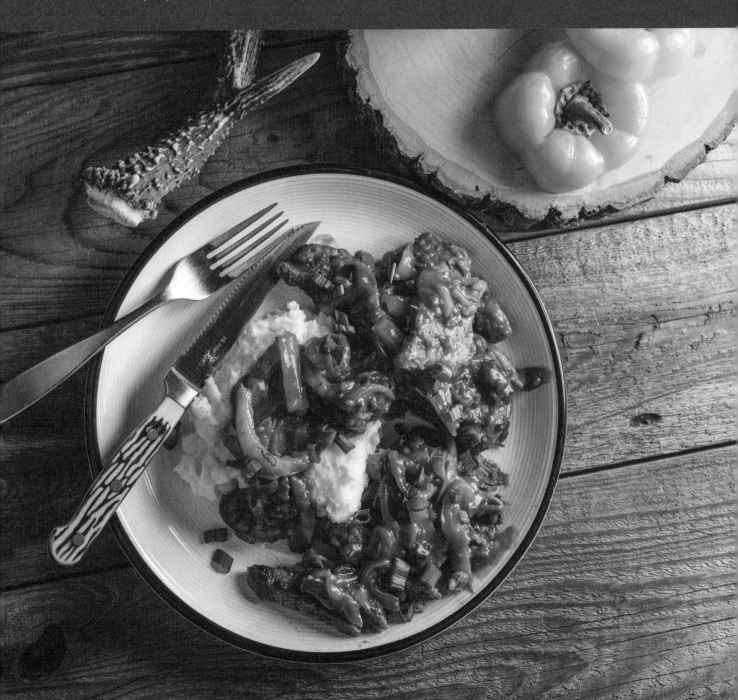

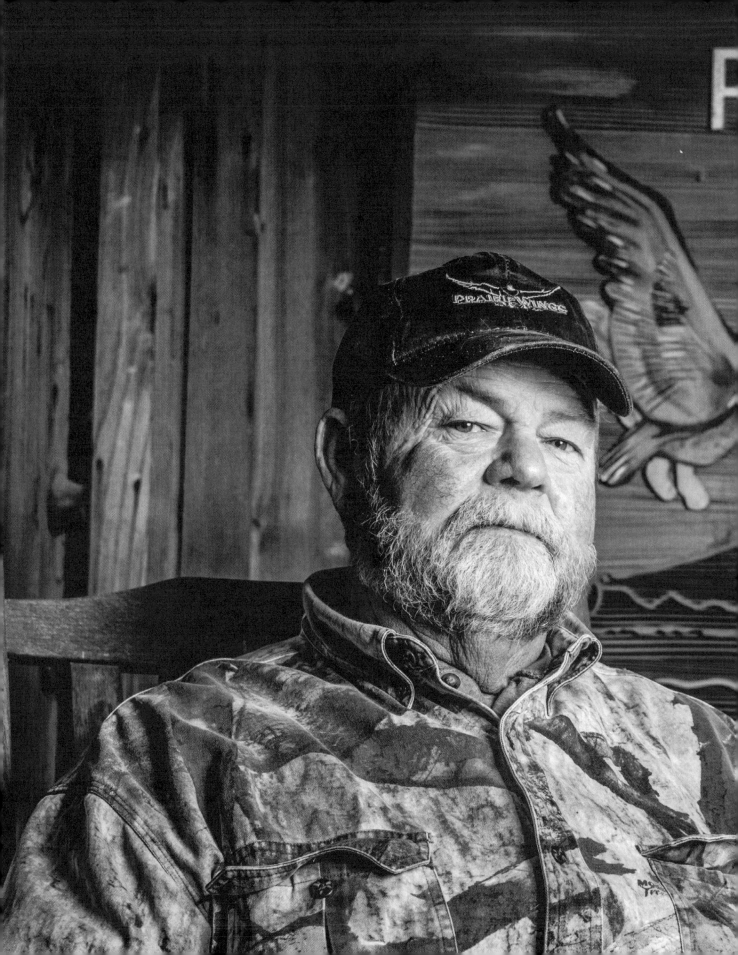

THE GREAT MR. BILLY BOGEY

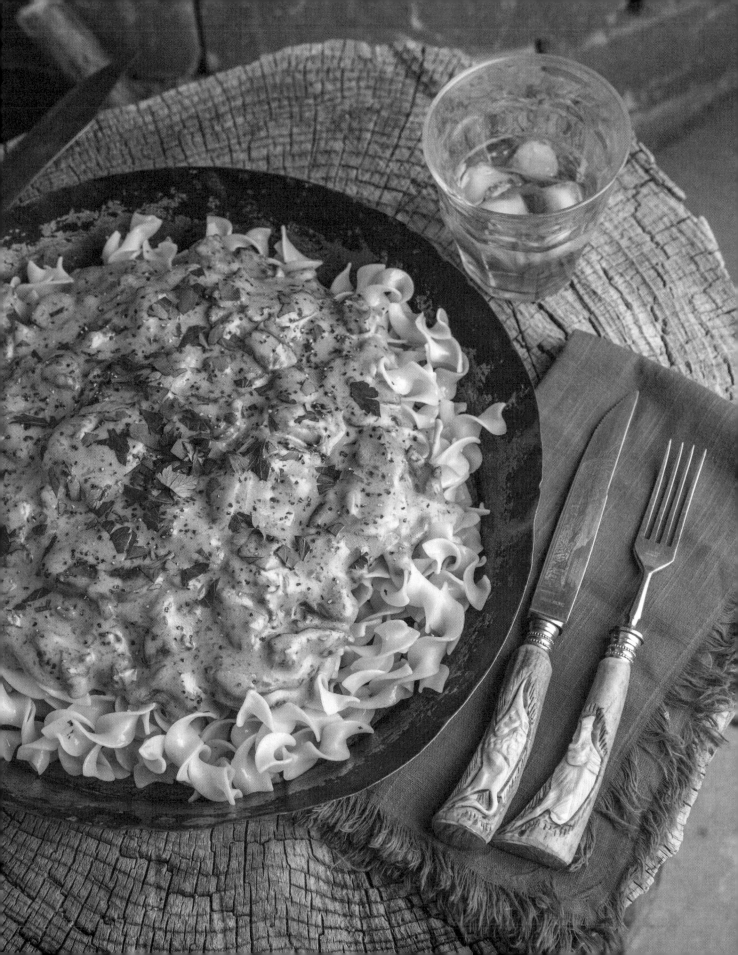

Wild Game Stroganoff

SERVES 4

This dish dates back to the late 1700s or early 1800s (depending on who you ask). The Russian aristocrat Count Stroganoff employed a French chef who's said to have added French mustard to his beef dish for seasoning and also used Russian sour cream. The chef named the concoction "Beef Stroganoff" after his benefactor.

When we were growing up, our moms might throw together a very simple version of this dish with a can of cream of mushroom soup, sliced onions, some ground beef, and a dollop of sour cream, served over egg noodles. There you have it: the quick and easy Americanized version of the Russian classic.

Fast-forward to present day and our friends Jim Rhea and Brad Forsythe use the basic framework of the Russian classic to dress up thinly sliced wild game. The lean meat is perfect for the rich, creamy sauce. Being Western hunters, they have used mule deer, antelope, and bighorn sheep to make this recipe and have served it over egg noodles, mashed potatoes, and French fries. Yes, French fries—they're also said to be traditional with stroganoff.

---

3 tablespoons unsalted butter

2 tablespoons olive oil

1½ pounds big game steaks, thinly sliced

Salt and ground black pepper to taste

2 shallots, finely chopped

12 ounces mushrooms, thinly sliced

2 tablespoons Dijon mustard

¼ cup brandy

1 cup sour cream

2 cups beef stock

1 cup heavy whipping cream

1 teaspoon Worcestershire sauce

2 garlic cloves, very finely chopped

Pinch smoked paprika

TO SERVE

Cooked egg noodles

Chopped fresh chives

Thinly sliced jalapeños (optional)

In a large cast-iron skillet, melt the butter with the olive oil over medium-high heat. Season the sliced meat with salt and pepper. When the skillet is hot, add the meat and brown it on both sides. Use tongs to transfer the meat to a plate, leaving the juices in the pan.

Add the shallots to the pan and cook for about 3 minutes, until they start to become translucent. Add the mushrooms and Dijon and stir for a minute or two.

continued

Meanwhile, heat the brandy in a small saucepan over medium heat until it begins to bubble at the edges (don't boil). Pour the hot brandy into the pan with the mushrooms and carefully ignite with a long match to flambé.

Once the flames subside, add the sour cream and beef stock and stir. Add the cream and Worcestershire sauce and stir again. Add the garlic and return the browned meat to the pan, along with any accumulated juices. Reduce the heat to medium and simmer for 10–15 minutes to thicken. Add a pinch of smoked paprika and continue to simmer to the desired thickness.

Serve the stroganoff over egg noodles and top with chopped chives and, if you like a bit of heat, sliced jalapeños.

Jim and Brad say: "Slice your game while the meat is partially frozen. It makes it much easier to get thin slices."

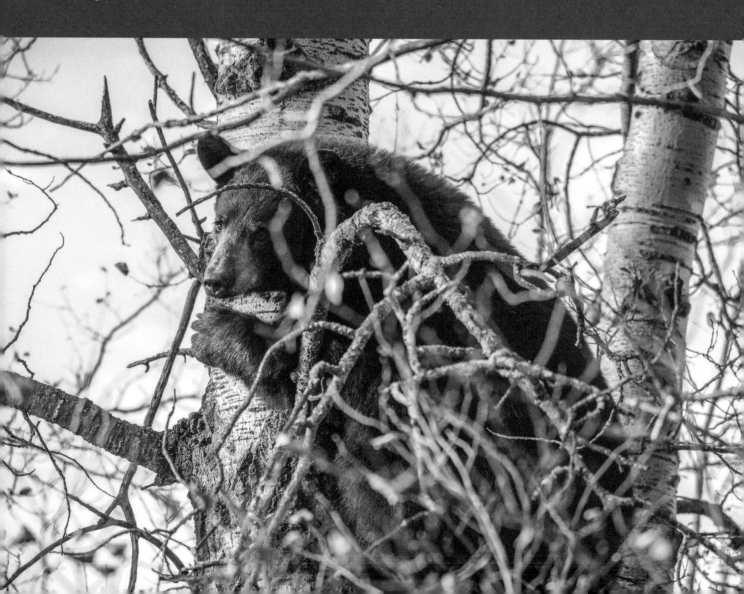

Bear Bourguignon

SERVES 5–6

Rihana Cary has been a friend of Chad Mendes for 5 or 6 years now. Chad met Rih through some mutual friends in the outdoor world. They had told him of this girl who would head out into the backcountry wilderness, by herself, with only a bow and a pack. She would live out there for days or weeks at a time and arrow giant bull elk, big bucks, or bear, then pack them out! Not going to lie, Chad half-expected her to have a screw loose—but after meeting Rihana for the first time, he was surprised to see how down to earth and kind she is. Rih's passion for the outdoors and living the Provider lifestyle shines through, and we are extremely excited to share a couple of her favorite recipes, including this hearty stew.

2–3 bacon slices, chopped

2 pounds bear or any game stew meat, cut into 2-inch cubes

1 large onion, chopped

5 garlic cloves, minced

3 cups wild game stock or beef stock

2 cups dry red wine

1 cup baby carrots

2 tablespoons all-purpose flour, divided

3 parsley sprigs

3 thyme sprigs

2 bay leaves

Salt and ground black pepper to taste

1 pound white or brown mushrooms, thickly sliced or quartered

TO SERVE

Mashed potatoes

Chopped fresh parsley

Preheat the oven to 300°F.

In a large Dutch oven, cook the bacon over medium heat for about 3 minutes, until it is lightly browned and crisp. Use a slotted spoon to transfer it to a plate lined with paper towels to drain, leaving the fat in the pan.

Add the bear meat to the pan (you may need to work in batches) and brown on all sides. Set it aside with the bacon.

Add the onion to the pan, reduce the heat to low, and cook for 3–4 minutes, until softened. Add the garlic and cook, stirring, for about 2 minutes, until fragrant.

continued

Return the bacon and bear to the pan, then follow with the stock, wine, carrots, 1 tablespoon of the flour, parsley, thyme, bay leaves, salt, and pepper. Stir well and make sure the meat is fully submerged in the liquid. Bring to a boil, then cover the Dutch oven and transfer to the oven. Bake for 1 hour.

Remove from the oven and stir in the mushrooms and remaining 1 tablespoon flour. Cover again and return to the oven for an additional 2 hours. Remove and discard the herb sprigs and bay leaves. Spoon the stew over mashed potatoes in individual bowls and sprinkle with parsley.

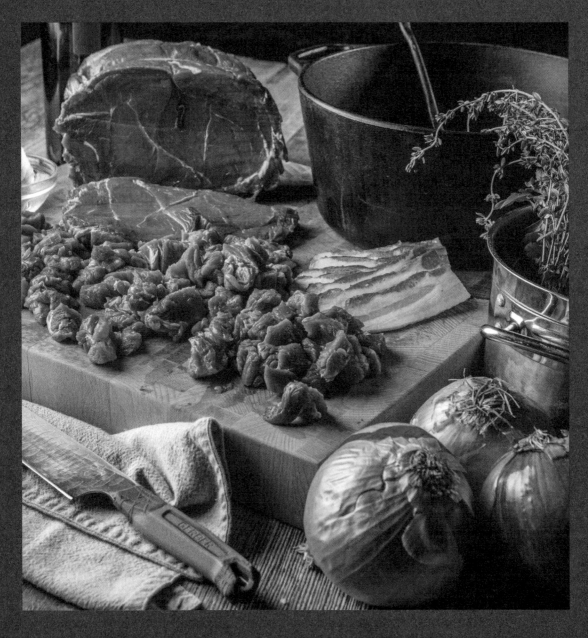

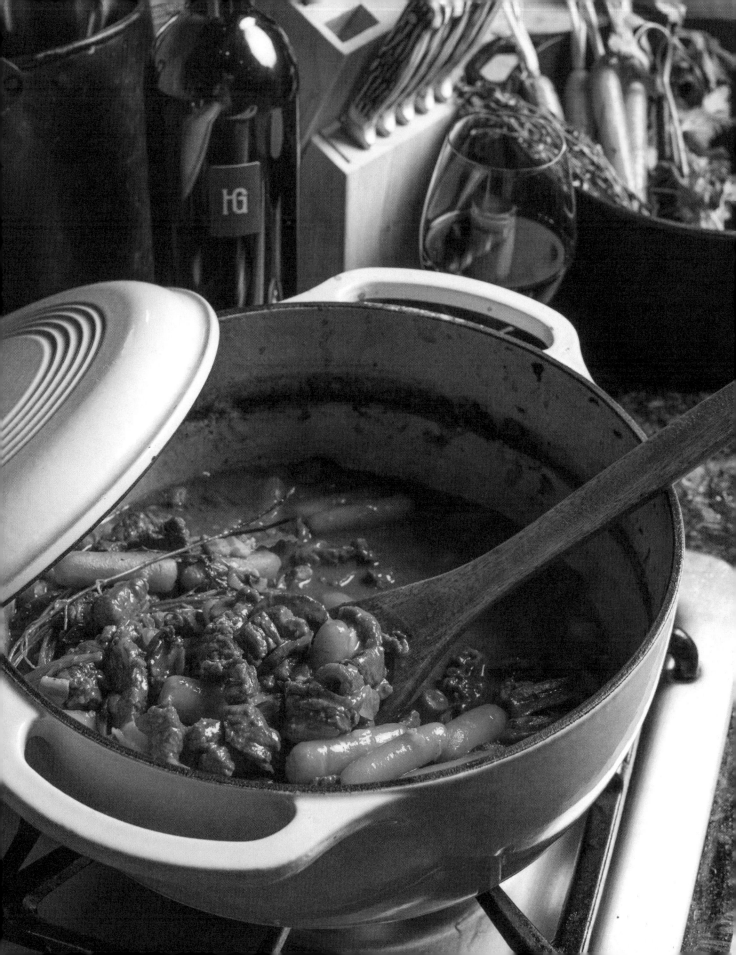

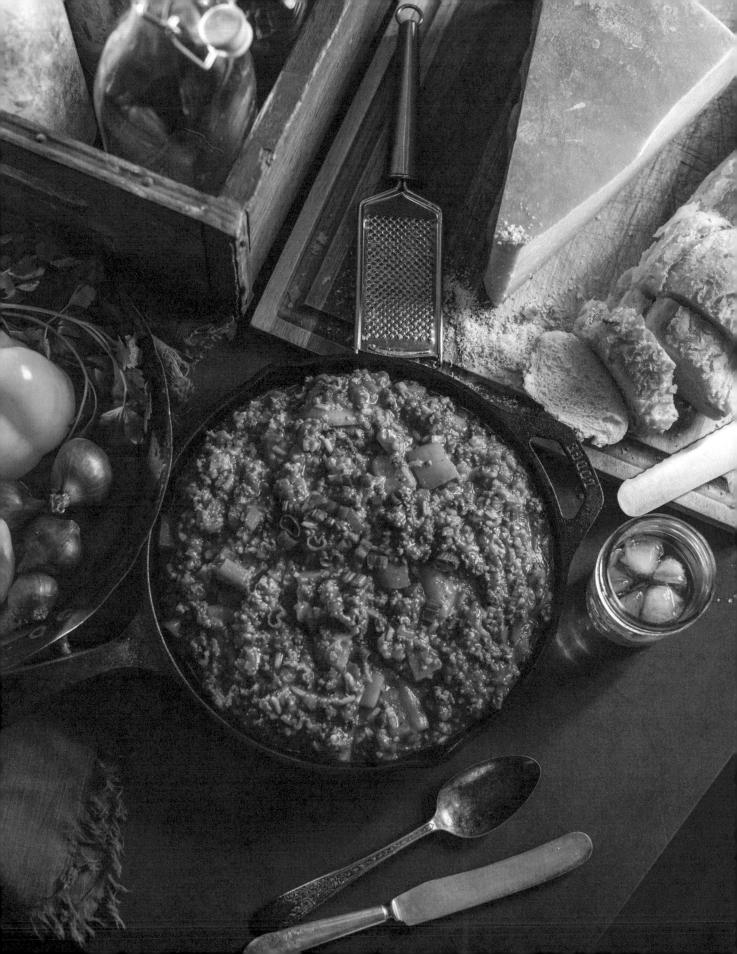

Cuban-Style Venison and Rice

SERVES 4

Chad Mendes says, "Visiting Abby's family, my in-laws, in the Midwest always means I'm about to gain a few pounds. The food is amazing and I always eat way more than I should! Her mom (whom we call Momma Judy) has a few amazing family recipes that have been passed down from generation to generation, including this simple but delicious dish." To save yourself some dishes, you can use Momma Judy's smart time-saver: use the emptied cans from the tomatoes to measure your water.

---

2 tablespoons olive oil

2 small onions, diced

1 pound ground venison

2 small bell peppers (any color), seeded and
  chopped

2 (14.5-ounce) cans petite diced tomatoes

3½ cups water

½ cup uncooked white rice

Salt to taste

In a large, deep frying pan, heat the olive oil over high heat. Add the onions and sauté until tender, 3–5 minutes. Add the ground venison and brown thoroughly. Add the bell peppers, tomatoes along with their juice, water, rice, and salt. Bring to a boil, then turn down to a simmer and cook, uncovered, until the rice is tender, about 15 minutes.

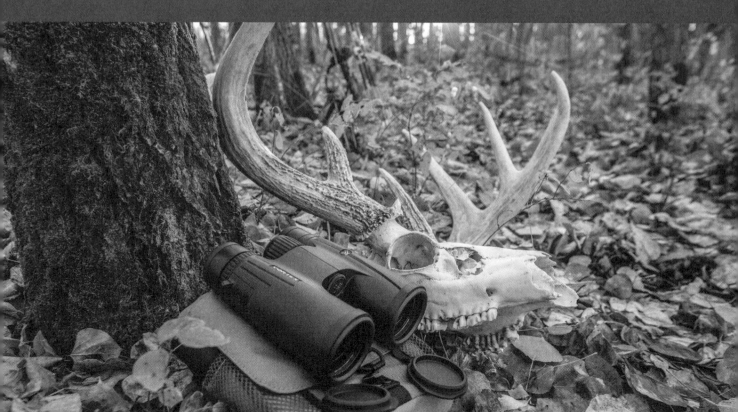

Spiced Bison Meatballs

SERVES 6-8

These meatballs are always a hit when we bring them to a tailgate or to a party for an appetizer.

---

1 pound ground bison

8 ounces bulk sweet or hot Italian sausage

2 large eggs

½ cup panko bread crumbs

⅓ cup grated parmesan cheese

⅓ cup finely chopped onion

⅓ cup finely chopped fresh parsley

3 garlic cloves, finely chopped

4 tablespoons The Provider Sonora Rub or your favorite spice rub

2 tablespoons olive oil, for stovetop cooking

In a large bowl, thoroughly mix all the ingredients, except the olive oil. Form the mixture into balls, using about 3 tablespoons for each.

ON A GRILL:
Preheat your grill (we use a Traeger) to 300°F. Place the meatballs directly on the grate and cook for 20–25 minutes, turning every few minutes, until cooked through. Or, if you want a crusty exterior, cook the meatballs on the grate for 15 minutes, then transfer them to a plate. Turn the grill to 350°F. Once the temperature is reached, return the meatballs to the grate and sear for about 1 minute on each side.

ON THE STOVETOP:
Heat the olive oil in a cast-iron skillet over medium heat. Add the meatballs and cook, turning the meatballs until browned on all sides and cooked through, about 20 minutes.

IN THE OVEN:
Preheat the oven to 350°F. Lightly grease a rimmed baking sheet. Place the meatballs on the sheet and bake for about 20 minutes, until cooked through. Or, if you want a crusty exterior, remove the meatballs after about 15 minutes, move the oven rack to the top position, and turn on the broiler to high. Return the meatballs to the oven and broil until the outside is crispy, about 5 minutes.

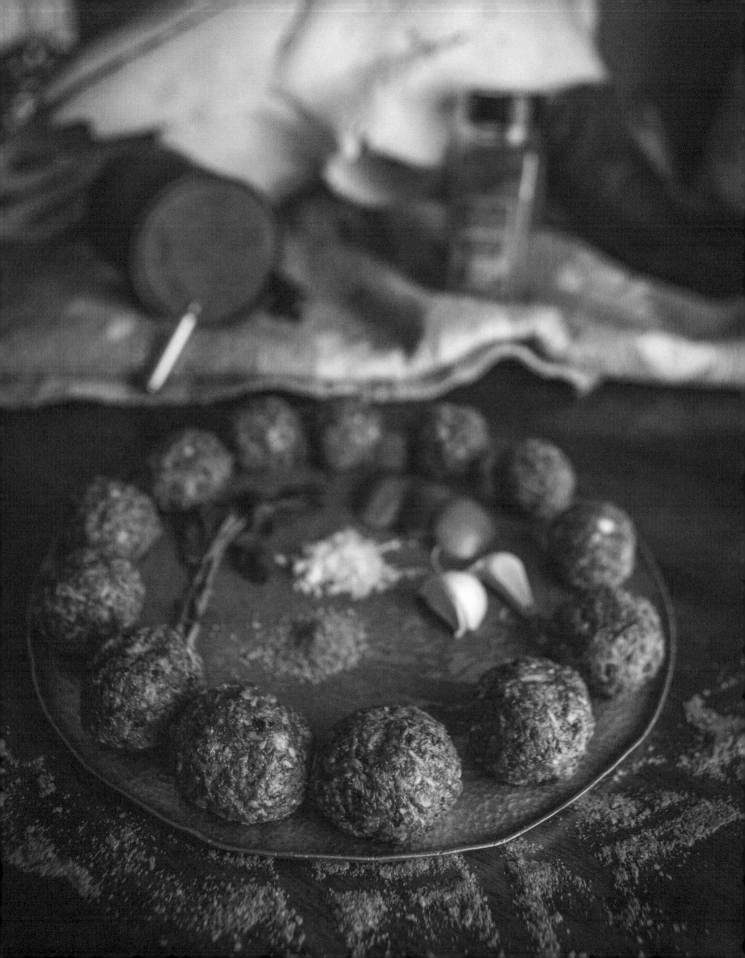

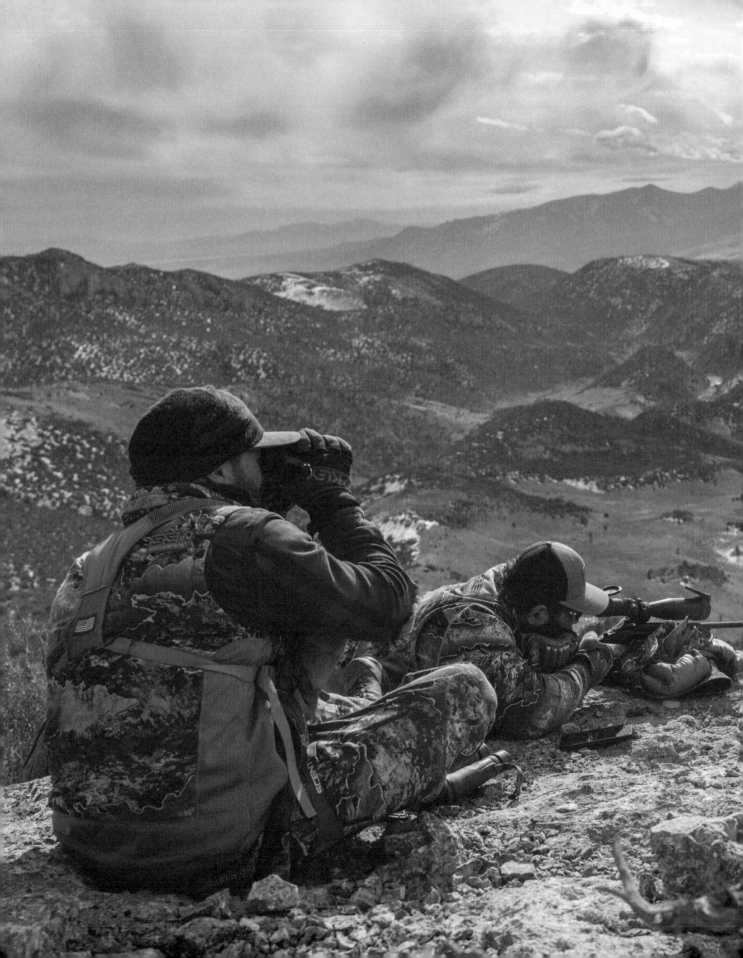

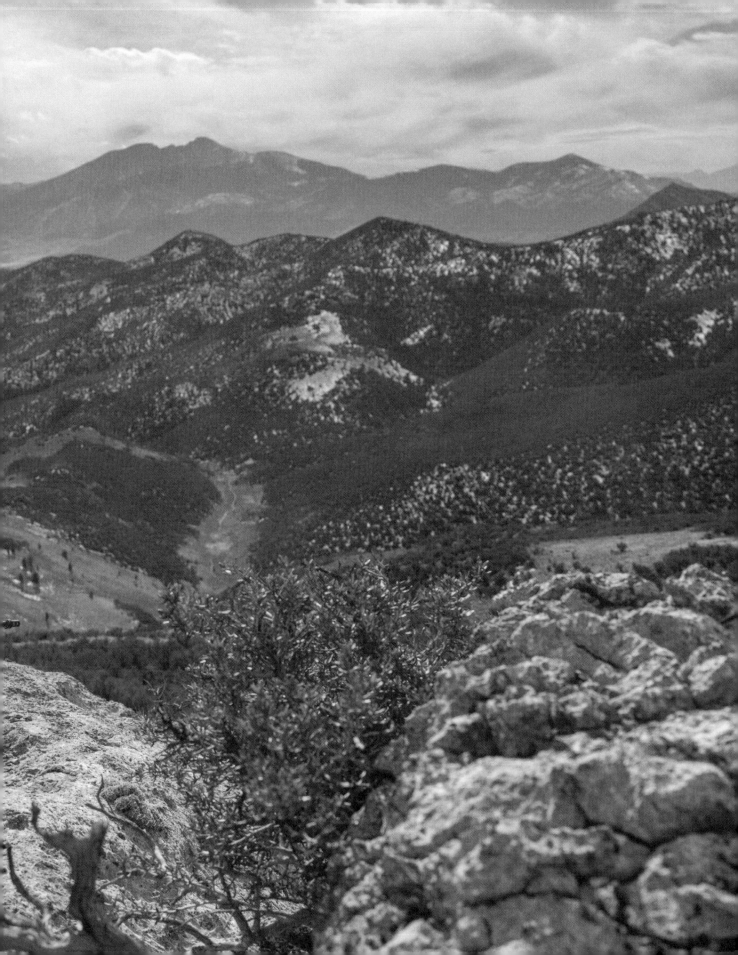

Antelope Backstrap Roulade

SERVES 4-6

This recipe is more on the advanced side, but we honestly feel anyone can master it! This unique dish is always a great way to feed your closest friends and family around the holiday season. The mix of flavors from the tender antelope backstraps, the pistachios, and of course the bacon will leave your guests speechless. We like this hearty roulade with the mild taste of antelope meat, though any backstrap will work. For larger animals like elk or moose, just cut about a 12-inch section. Pair with a full-bodied red wine.

---

1 whole antelope backstrap

1 tablespoon olive oil

½ sweet onion, chopped

½ cup chopped mushrooms

2 cups roughly chopped spinach

2 garlic cloves, minced

2 bacon slices

¼ cup cream cheese

3 tablespoons crushed pistachios

¼ cup The Provider Drop Tine or Crosshairs Rub or your favorite spice rub, plus more as needed

---

Preheat your grill (we use a Traeger) to 450°F with a cast-iron skillet inside.

Carefully butterfly the backstrap, leaving a strip of meat connecting the halves. Cover with a sheet of plastic wrap. With a meat mallet, lightly pound and flatten it to an even thickness (¼–½ inch). Remove the plastic wrap.

In a large frying pan, heat the olive oil over medium-high heat. Sauté the onion and mushrooms until tender, 5–10 minutes. Add the spinach and garlic and cook until the spinach is wilted. Transfer the vegetables to a bowl.

In the same pan, cook the bacon until crispy. Transfer the bacon to a plate lined with a paper towel, reserving the fat in the pan.

Smear the cream cheese evenly on one side of the meat. Place the bacon on top, making sure to cover the entire length of the meat. Add the vegetable mixture next. Sprinkle the crushed pistachios on top. Roll the backstrap into a cylinder and tie every 3–4 inches with butcher's twine. With a basting brush, coat the entire outside of the roll with the reserved bacon grease and season all over with the spice rub. Start with ¼ cup and see if you need more.

Place the roulade in the hot cast-iron skillet and close the grill. Rotate the roulade every 2–4 minutes until cooked through, 15–20 minutes total. Transfer to a cutting board, loosely cover with aluminum foil, and let rest for 10 minutes. Cut the roulade into slices about 1 inch thick and serve.

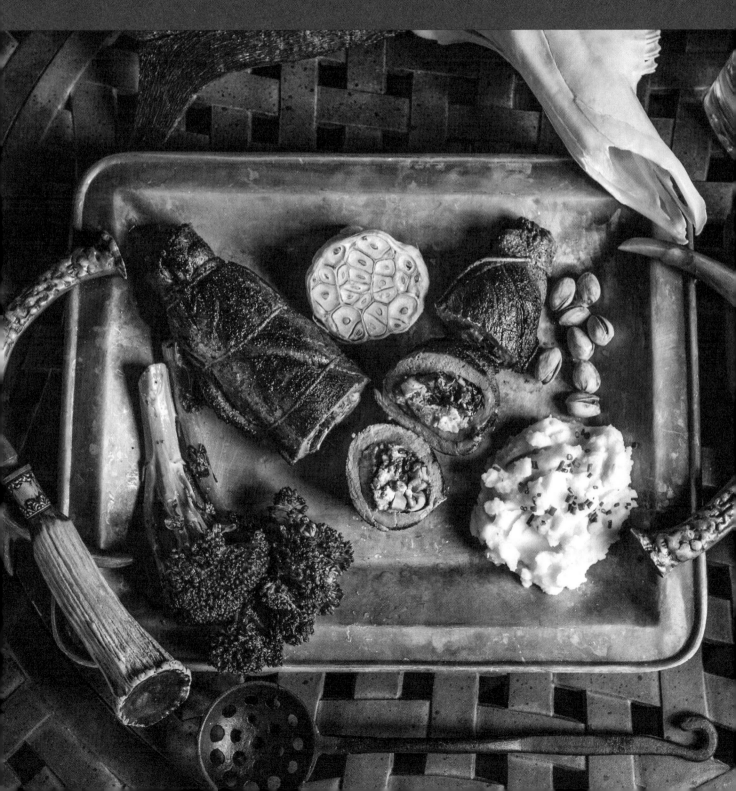

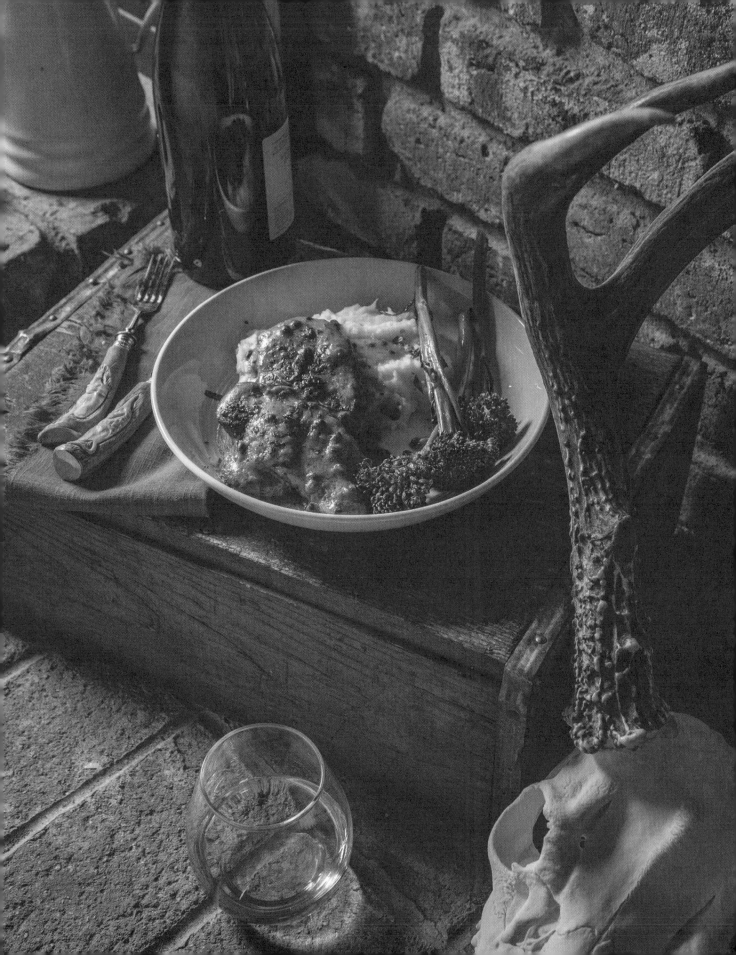

Venison Piccata

SERVES 4-5

This is hands down our favorite thing to do with backstraps! The tenderness of the meat and the flavorful sauce will make you think you're eating at a five-star restaurant. This recipe works great with any wild game loin or any other mild, tender cut of meat. Serve with creamy polenta or mashed potatoes.

½ venison backstrap (about 2 pounds)

½ cup plus 1½ tablespoons all-purpose flour, divided

Grated zest of 1 lemon

Salt and ground black pepper to taste

3 tablespoons olive oil

4 tablespoons (½ stick) unsalted butter

1 cup chicken stock

½ cup dry white wine

1½ tablespoons lemon juice

¼ cup capers, drained

3 tablespoons chopped fresh parsley

Cut the venison into 1-inch medallions. Cover with a sheet of plastic wrap and pound to ½-inch thickness.

In a bowl, combine ½ cup of the flour, the lemon zest, and a few pinches each of salt and pepper. Dredge the venison pieces in the flour mixture to evenly coat, then shake off the excess.

In a large cast-iron skillet, heat the olive oil over medium-high heat. Sear the venison pieces for 1–2 minutes on each side, working in batches if needed to not crowd the skillet. Transfer to a plate and cover loosely with aluminum foil to keep warm.

In the same skillet, melt the butter and whisk in the remaining 1½ tablespoons flour until smooth; cook this roux until lightly browned, 1–2 minutes. Gradually stir in the chicken stock, whisking after each addition until smooth. Add the white wine, lemon juice, and capers. Simmer for about 3 minutes, whisking occasionally, until the sauce has thickened slightly. Return the venison pieces to the pan and simmer for 2–4 minutes, until the venison is done to your liking. Since venison is very lean, take care not to overcook. Top with the parsley and serve.

Wild Boar Sausage and Goat Cheese Pasta

SERVES 5-6

Being part Italian, Chad Mendes has always enjoyed creating pasta dishes. After years of the standard red sauce creations, he decided to think outside the box a bit. Roasted red peppers and goat cheese have always gone so well together with crackers and wine. Why not in a pasta? Throw in a little wild boar sausage and bingo! This creation immediately became a favorite pasta dish and one his friends often request for get-together dinners.

---

1 pound angel hair pasta

6 tablespoons olive oil, divided

½ white onion, chopped

3 cups chopped mushrooms

2 garlic cloves, minced

Salt and ground black pepper to taste

1 pound bulk wild boar sausage or any Italian sausage

¼ cup balsamic vinegar

1 cup sliced roasted red peppers

3 ounces goat cheese, crumbled

Bring a large pot of water to a boil and add the angel hair pasta and 2 tablespoons of the olive oil. Cook the pasta according to the package directions. Drain, return the pasta to the pot, and set aside.

Heat another 2 tablespoons olive oil in a large frying pan over medium-high heat. Add the onion, mushrooms, and garlic and cook until soft. Season with salt and pepper. Add the boar sausage and cook, breaking it up with a fork to make crumbles, until cooked through.

Add the meat and vegetables to the pot with the cooked pasta. Stir in the balsamic vinegar, red peppers, goat cheese, and remaining 2 tablespoons olive oil. Toss to mix everything together and serve immediately.

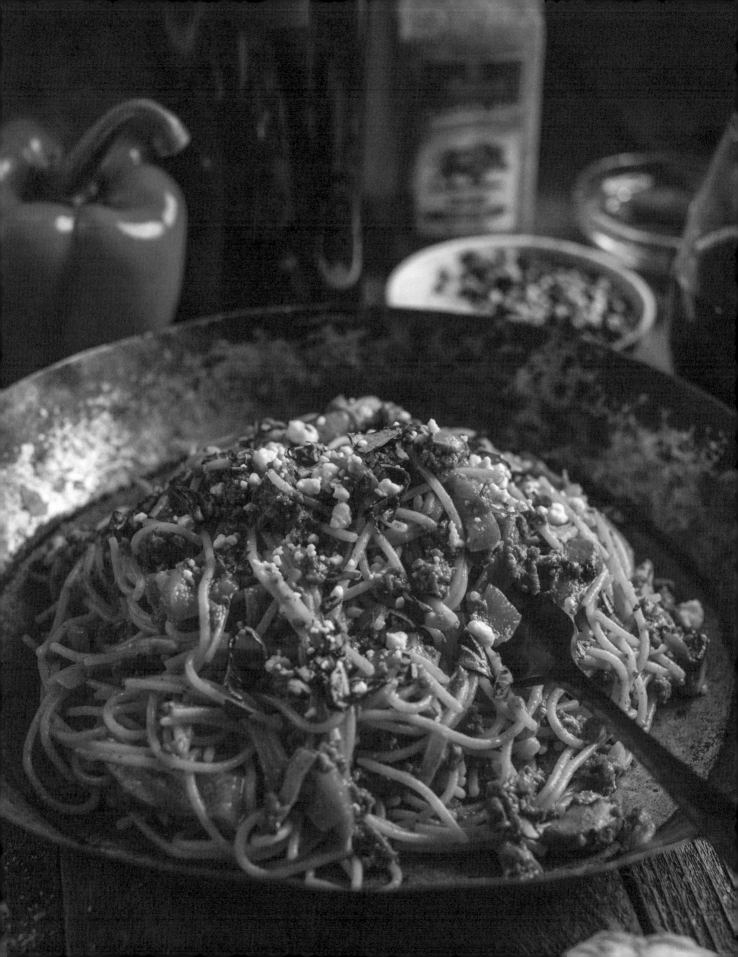

Ole Betsy and the Wild Boar Hunt

Chad Mendes

My good friend Mike was the head guide on an absolutely beautiful ranch down in the Central Valley in California. It was loaded with wild pigs, monster bucks, and tons of upland game. I would come down pretty regularly to load up on wild pork to live off of for my training camps. One pig hunt will probably never be topped in my book. It was right after I graduated from Cal Poly and began my MMA career up in Sacramento.

At the front entrance to the ranch, the owner had two big irrigated pastures that he ran cattle in. Right in the middle of the two pastures was a big creek with thick brush and big oaks—perfect for wild pigs. They had water, amazing feed, and great cover for bedding. Every morning and evening you could expect to see multiple groups of pigs out there, often over 30 at a time! With so many cattle in those pastures, though, it was tough to use a rifle, and the grass wasn't tall enough to sneak into bow range.

One day I figured out the solution. I sat down with a huge flat of cardboard and cut out the shape of a cow. I painted it black like the cattle that were out there and cut two flap windows right in the middle. We fondly called her Ole Betsy. My dad decided he would give it a shot first. We headed out for the evening hunt. As we pulled up to the gate, we immediately saw a giant boar out feeding solo. Game time! We got all our stuff in order, and my dad and Mike started to sneak in with the cardboard cow. I decided to stay back on the creek tree line to film, but I brought my bow just in case.

The boar would look up every once in a while, and my dad and Mike (and Ole Betsy) would freeze. As soon as he went back to feeding, they slowly started creeping again. After about 15 minutes of stalking in, they were finally in range. Thirty-five yards! Mike held Ole Betsy and opened the window in the middle. My dad drew back and released. The arrow went right over the boar's back! He jumped but thankfully had no clue what just happened. After about 30 seconds of looking around, he went back to feeding. My dad pulled back and released again. This time it was too low! The boar jumped again but still didn't know what was happening. My dad pulled back and released one more arrow, this time connecting right behind the shoulder. The boar took off in a dead sprint—directly toward me! I dropped the camera and knocked an arrow as quick as I could. I knew I was between him and his goal, the line of trees. At about 40 yards out, the boar realized what I was and began to charge me. I drew my bow and stood my ground. At 10 yards I released my arrow and the boar slid to my feet! Up close you could see he what a giant he was, with 4-inch razor blades for teeth. My arrow had hit him right between the eyes, killing him instantly. My heart was about to beat out of my chest and my hands were shaking. Who knows what would have happened if my arrow had missed?

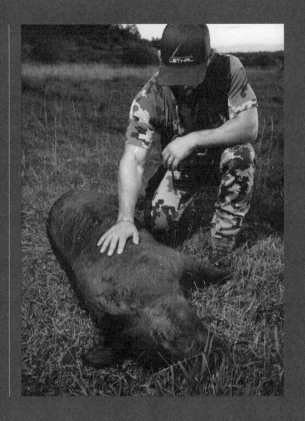

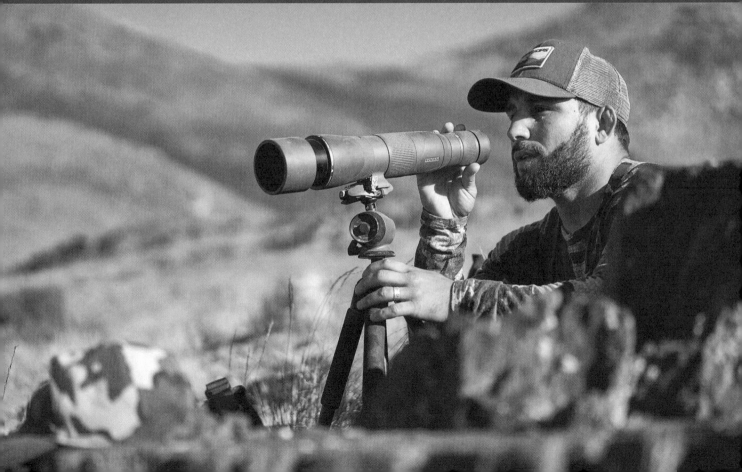

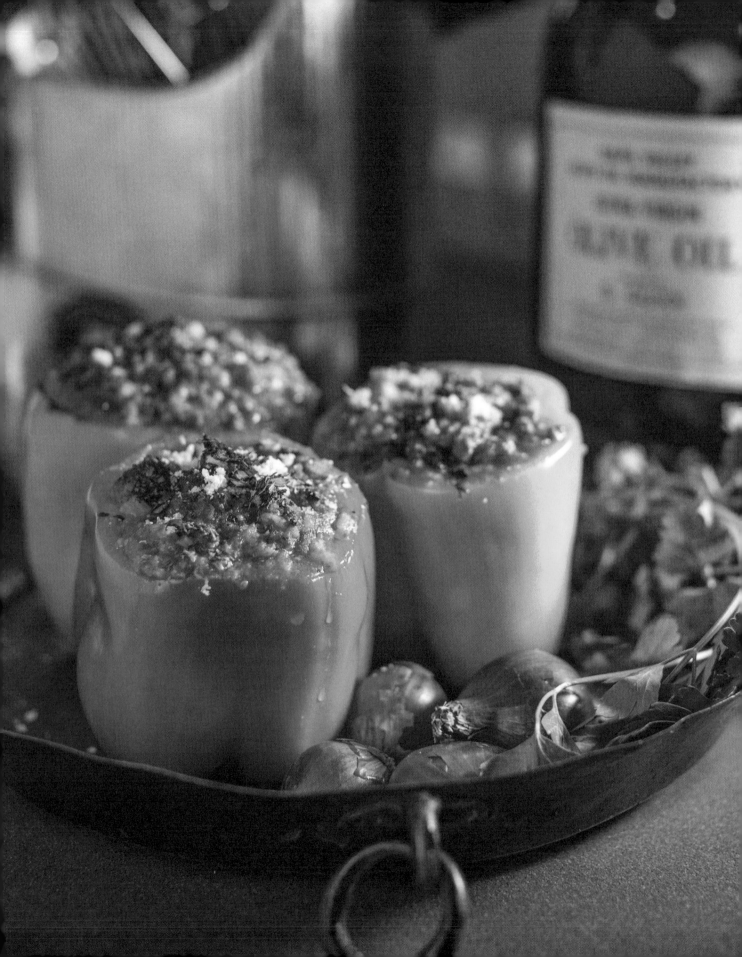

Ground Elk Stuffed Bell Peppers

SERVES 4

This recipe came about during one of our garden bell pepper harvests. We were trying to find unique ways to use them and this was one of our favorites! It's a super simple, healthy, and delicious dinner.

---

4 large bell peppers (any color)

2 tablespoons olive oil

½ sweet onion, diced

3 garlic cloves, minced

1 pound ground elk

Salt and ground black pepper to taste

1 (14.5-ounce) can diced fire-roasted tomatoes

2 cups cooked brown or white rice

⅓ cup feta cheese crumbles or any shredded cheese

¼ cup chopped fresh cilantro

Preheat your grill (we use a Traeger) or oven to 400°F.

Cut around the stem on the top of each bell pepper to open up the top. Remove and toss the seeds and the stem. Make a thin slice off the bottom of any pepper that won't stand upright on its own.

In a large frying pan, heat the olive oil over medium-high heat and sauté the onion and garlic until tender, 3–5 minutes. Add the ground elk and cook, breaking it into small pieces as it browns. Season with salt and pepper while it cooks. When the meat is browned, add the fire-roasted tomatoes with their juice. Mix and simmer for 5 minutes, or until the mixture is as thick as you like.

Add the rice, cheese, and cilantro and mix together.

Fill the bell peppers with the mixture. Stand the bell peppers in a cast-iron skillet or baking dish and transfer it to your grill or oven. Cook until the peppers start getting soft, about 15 minutes. Remove and serve.

The Money Elk Burger

SERVES 4

Here's another great recipe for all that ground meat! Who doesn't like a good juicy burger? Chad Mendes often makes these burgers for the family and they absolutely love the flavor combination. The fried egg and avocado mash make this burger next level!

---

1 avocado, peeled and pitted

1 teaspoon garlic powder

Salt to taste

1 pound ground elk (20% fat added is ideal)

1½ tablespoons The Provider Crosshairs Rub
  or your favorite spice rub

1 tablespoon yellow mustard

2 squirts hot sauce (we like Tabasco)

3–4 drops liquid smoke

4 slices pepper Jack cheese

TO SERVE

Neutral vegetable oil, for greasing the pan

4 large eggs

Potato buns

Mayonnaise

Barbecue sauce

Green leaf lettuce

Tomato slices

Sliced dill pickles

Preheat your grill (we use a Traeger) to 450°F with a cast-iron skillet inside.

In a small bowl, mash and mix the avocado, garlic powder, and salt. Cover and chill until you're ready to serve.

In a large bowl, combine the ground elk, spice rub, mustard, hot sauce, and liquid smoke. Try not to overwork the meat. Form 4 patties about an inch bigger than the buns since they will shrink a bit when grilled. Make an indention in the middle of the patties to keep them from plumping in the center.

Once the grill and skillet are hot, place the patties in the skillet. Let the patties brown and sear well before flipping, about 3 minutes on each side. They should feel firm but not hard. With about a minute left of cooking on the second side, add a slice of pepper Jack cheese to each patty.

Once the patties are done, generously oil a large frying pan and fry the eggs over medium heat to your desired doneness. Meanwhile, toast the buns on the grill.

Top both halves of each bun with mayo and barbecue sauce. On the bottom bun, stack your lettuce, tomato, and pickles. Top that with your cheesy patty. Next add your fried egg. Spread the avocado mash on the top bun, close them up, and enjoy!

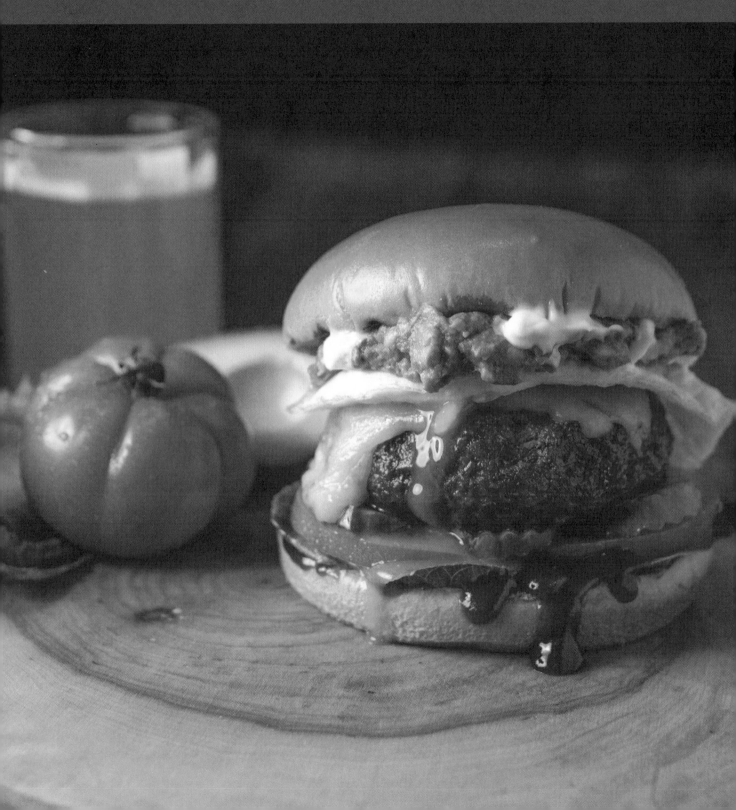

My First Chance at a Bull

Clint Belding

The alarm clock chirped in the dark of the night. It would have been an unwelcome disruption to a normal night's sleep, but this was no normal morning. I was up several minutes before the alarm in anticipation of what the day might bring. My first task was to make sure the team was up and out of bed. The second task was to get the burner lit to warm the wall tent and, equally important, get the camp coffee brewing.

It was the seventh morning of my 16-year-old son's Nevada bull elk hunt. We spent the first two days in search of a good bull that we had found a few weeks earlier while scouting. After two long days on the prowl, with tired legs and eyes, we couldn't turn him up. With the help of great optics, I was able to spot a group of elk a long ways off. The team agreed that the amount of horn that we could pick up through the spotting scope at that distance was worth getting a closer look.

We were able to close the distance by truck, but to get a better look, it would require a good afternoon hike. Three of us took off on the trek, leaving behind two spotters. As we approached the area of thick juniper and piñion pines where we figured the herd to be, we climbed a steep face to gain a vantage point. Within a few hours, the distant mooing of cows could be heard. It's quite an experience to hear a group of animals before you actually see them. What happened over the next hour would make for a great campfire story that night. A herd of no less than a hundred elk began to cross a ridge 500 yards in front of us. We began the task of trying to pick out the herd bull among the massive group. After watching and hearing dozens of cows and half a dozen satellite bulls pass through the trees, the unmistakable body size and 7-by-6 frame of the herd bull emerged. Steep terrain, one hundred-plus noses, and the wrong wind prevented a late-afternoon stalk. This disappointment was countered by the sheer beauty of watching a massive herd of elk feed across the ridge lit brightly by the warming sun.

Over the next three days, we hiked and glassed as hard as we could. We were fortunate enough to find the herd each day. Unfortunately, we could never get any closer than the 500 yards that separated us from the big bull that first day.

The fifth day of the hunt would prove pivotal. We set out in the dark to hike to a vantage point that we thought would give us a good chance at finally putting a stalk on our wily adversary. This game of cat and mouse would again favor the big bull, as we were not able to find him. After a few hours of glassing the vast mountain, we hiked back down the ridge to regroup. Our intuition told us that since we hadn't spotted the large group in the area where we thought they would be, there was a decent chance they might have circled back around to the area where they were first spotted. After the better part of a week chasing this bull around, we finally had a stroke of luck. The elk were spotted high on a ridge bedded down in the early afternoon.

With the wind direction to our advantage, we put together a plan to close the distance and see if my son could get in a position to take a shot. On the last night of our hunt and with little time to spare before sunset, it was now or never. As we were making our way up the ridge, a group of about 20 elk, including the big bull, got up from their beds and started feeding toward a secluded water hole. This ended up helping us out tremendously because we were between the elk and the water source. Sometimes with hunting, it's better to be lucky than good!

My son was able to harvest his first bull elk with as ethical a shot as you could hope to take from 178 yards. The team worked for the next four hours in the dark field dressing and quartering the massive bull. Many nights since have been spent around the dinner table with family and friends reminiscing about the epic hunt while enjoying a burger or a choice cut of venison backstrap from a genuine trophy.

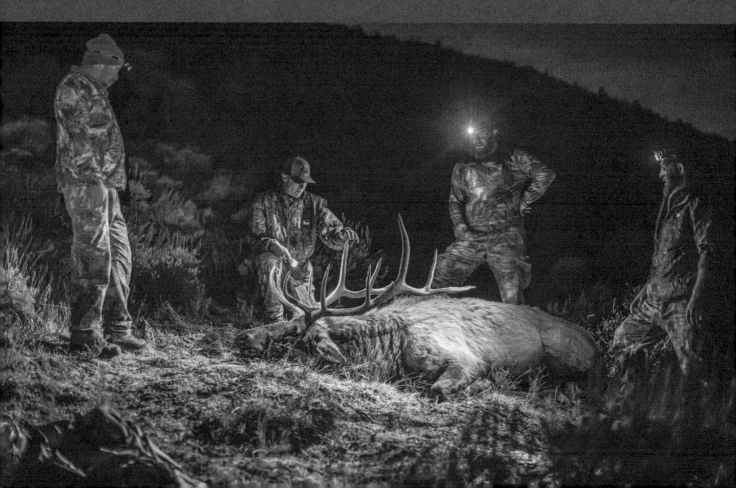

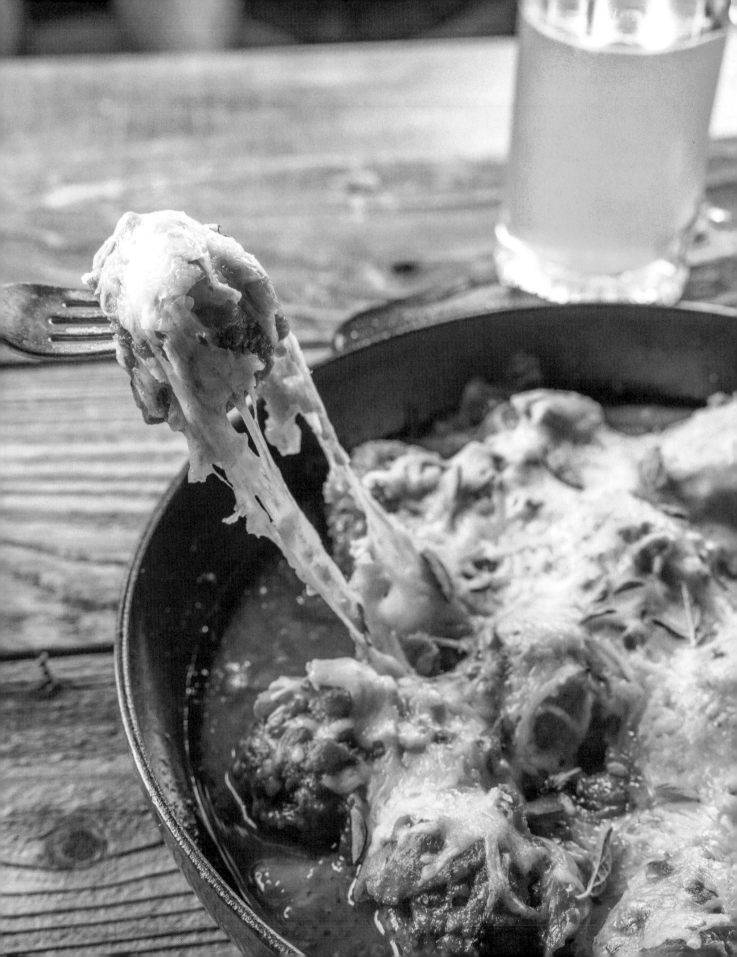

Elk Pizza Meatballs

SERVES 4

With all the flavors of a pizza wrapped up in a tender meatball, these are always a huge hit at any get-together!

---

3 tablespoons Italian bread crumbs

¼ cup milk

1 tablespoon olive oil

½ white onion, finely chopped

1 pound bulk Italian elk sausage

1 large egg

⅓ cup chopped fresh parsley

2 garlic cloves, minced

2 tablespoons grated parmesan cheese

1 (24-ounce) jar marinara sauce

8 ounces fresh mozzarella cheese, sliced

In a bowl, soak the bread crumbs in the milk for 20 minutes.

Meanwhile, heat the olive oil in a large skillet over medium-high heat. Sauté the onion until tender, 10–15 minutes.

In a mixing bowl, combine the sausage, onion, bread crumb mixture, egg, parsley, garlic, and parmesan cheese. Mix well, cover, and refrigerate for at least 1 hour and up to overnight.

Preheat your grill (we use a Traeger) or oven to 450°F.

Lightly grease a 2-quart casserole dish. Form the meat into balls about 1½ inches in diameter and place in the dish. Pour the marinara sauce over the meatballs.

Place in the grill or oven for 15 minutes. Add the mozzarella cheese slices to cover all the meatballs. Cook for another 5–10 minutes, until the cheese is melted and bubbly. Let cool for about 10 minutes before serving.

Wild Boar Quiche

SERVES 6

This recipe, courtesy of Momma Judy Raines, can easily be customized to your liking. You can add any veggies you wish—simply sauté them along with the sausage and onion.

---

8 ounces bulk wild boar breakfast sausage

⅓ cup diced onion

½ cup milk

½ cup mayonnaise

3 large eggs

1 tablespoon cornstarch

¾ cup shredded cheddar cheese

¾ cup shredded Swiss cheese

½ teaspoon salt

½ teaspoon ground black pepper

1 (9-inch) pie crust (store-bought or homemade)

Preheat your oven or grill (we use a Traeger) to 350°F.

Heat a large frying pan over medium-high heat. Brown the sausage and onion, breaking up the meat up with a spatula, until the onion is soft and the sausage is cooked through.

In a large mixing bowl, combine the milk, mayo, eggs, and cornstarch and beat until smooth. Add the sausage and onion mixture, cheeses, salt, and pepper. Mix well.

Place the pie crust in a pie plate. (Skip this if you're using a premade crust with a foil tray; just bake the quiche in that.) Pour the egg filling into the crust. Bake for 35–45 minutes, until a knife inserted into the middle comes out dry.

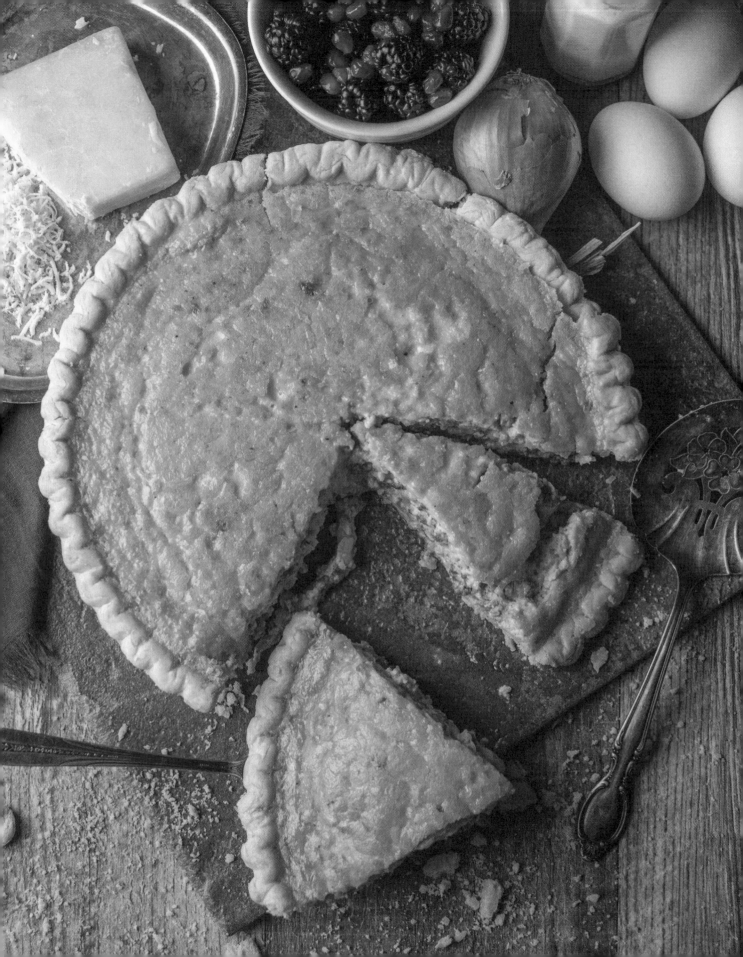

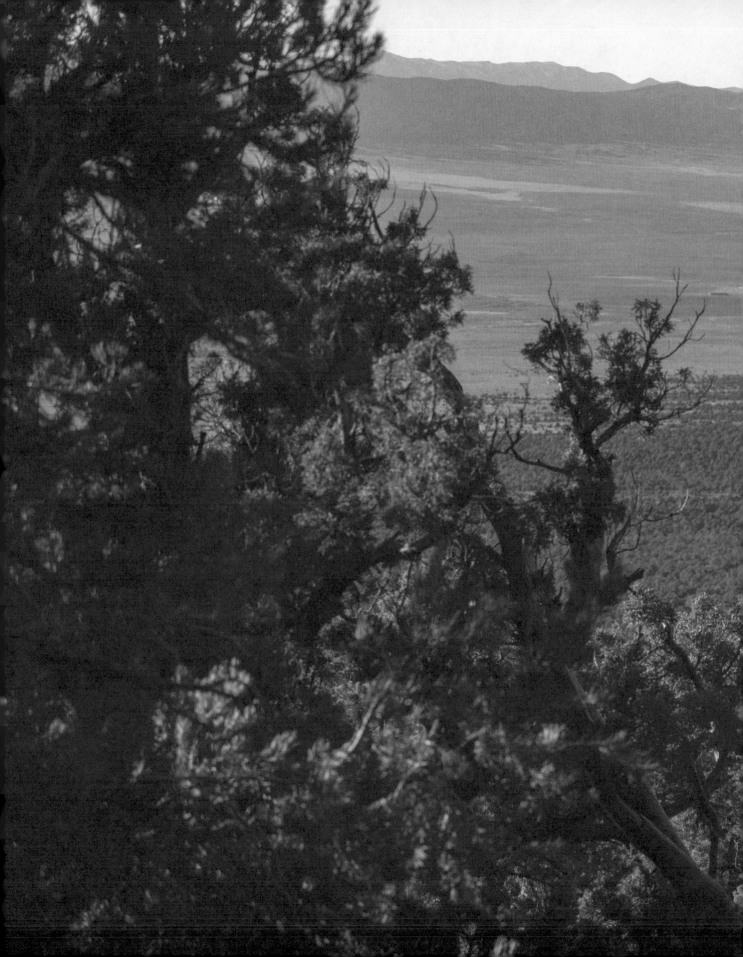

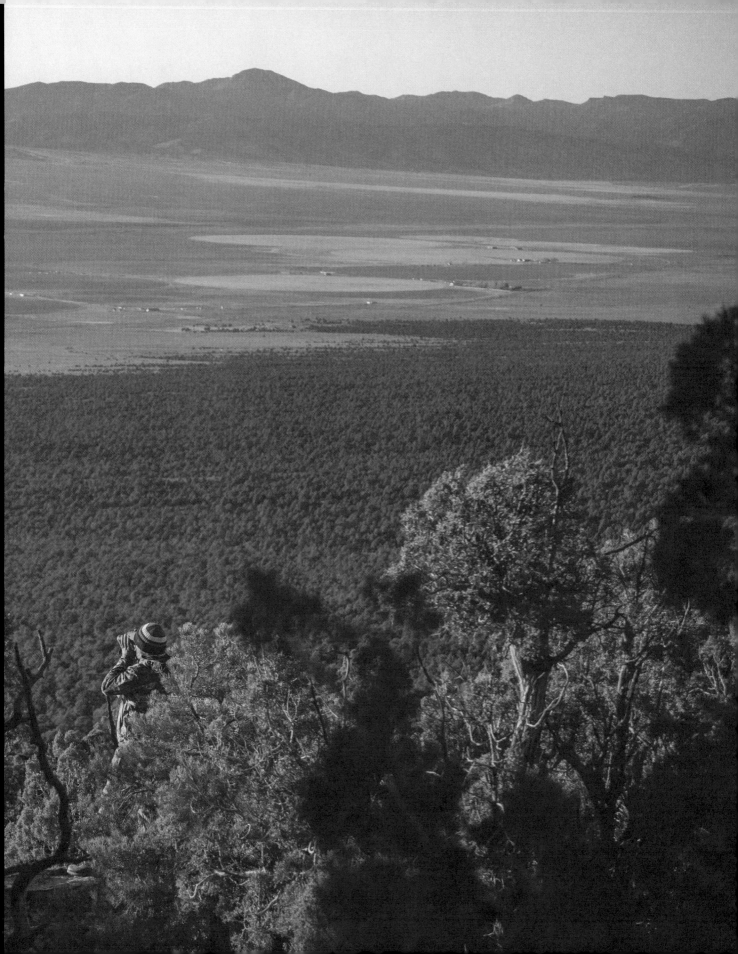

Mama Cobb's Deer-Stuffed Cabbage

SERVES 6

Brent Cobb is a master of words and lyrics. His songs trace his life from childhood to becoming one of the most popular songwriters in all of music. He often writes and sings of his family and everything that was part of his Georgia upbringing, and food is naturally ingrained throughout. This stuffed cabbage dish, courtesy of Brent, is straight Southern comfort food that will make you want to hug your brothers and kiss your babies!

---

1 large head green cabbage, cored

1½ pounds ground venison

¾ cup uncooked white rice

1 medium onion, chopped

½ green bell pepper, seeded and chopped

1 teaspoon garlic powder

½ teaspoon salt

¼ teaspoon ground black pepper

2 teaspoons Worcestershire sauce

2 (10.75-ounce) cans condensed tomato soup

Water, as needed

Preheat the oven to 350°F.

Bring a large pot of water to a boil. Immerse the head of cabbage in the boiling water for several minutes. Peel off the leaves as they soften and place in a colander to cool.

In a bowl, combine the venison, rice, onion, bell pepper, garlic powder, salt, black pepper, and Worcestershire sauce. Scoop up a small fistful of the meat mixture and place on a large cabbage leaf. Roll up the leaf beginning at the thick end, pushing in the sides as you as you roll. Place the roll seam-side down in a large roasting pan. Repeat with the remaining meat mixture and cabbage leaves; you should get about 12 rolls.

continued

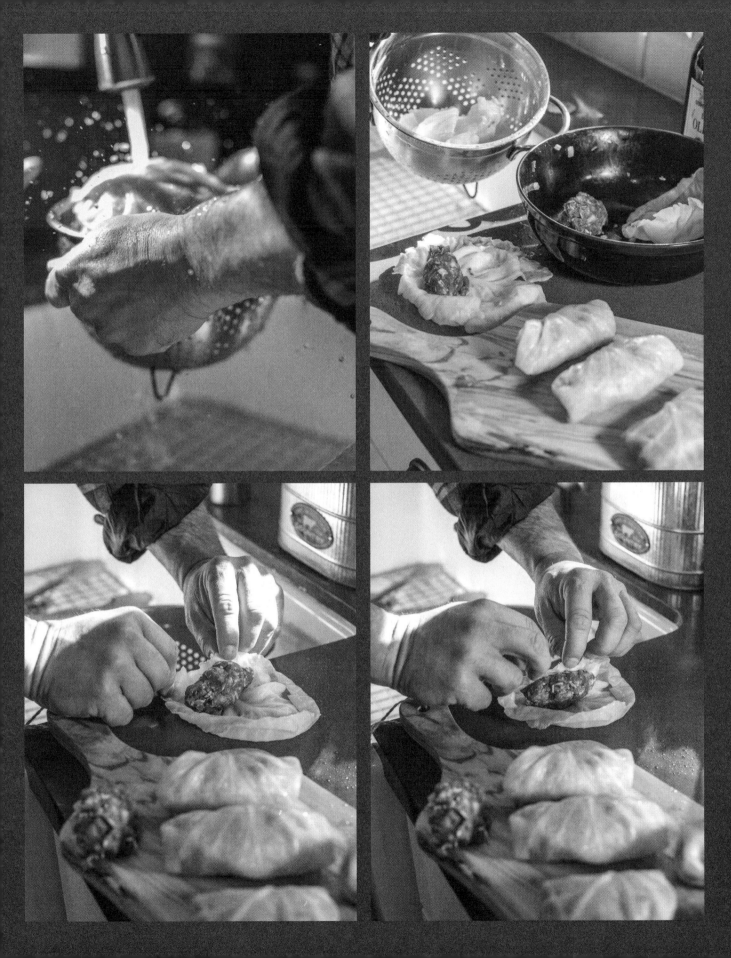

Chop up the remaining cabbage leaves, including the ones that are too small to roll, and scatter on top of the stuffed cabbage rolls.

Add the tomato soup and enough water to just cover.

Cover the pan with a lid or aluminum foil and bake for about 3½ hours, until the rice and meat are cooked. You may need to keep pressing the cabbage rolls down into the juice as they cook.

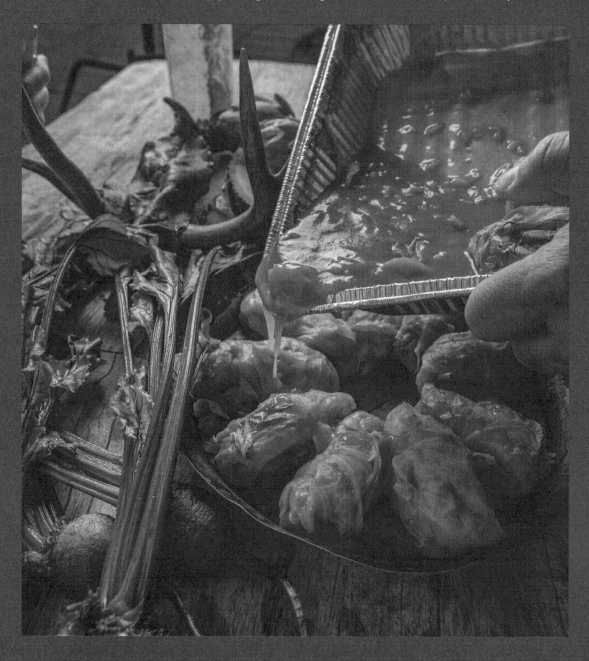

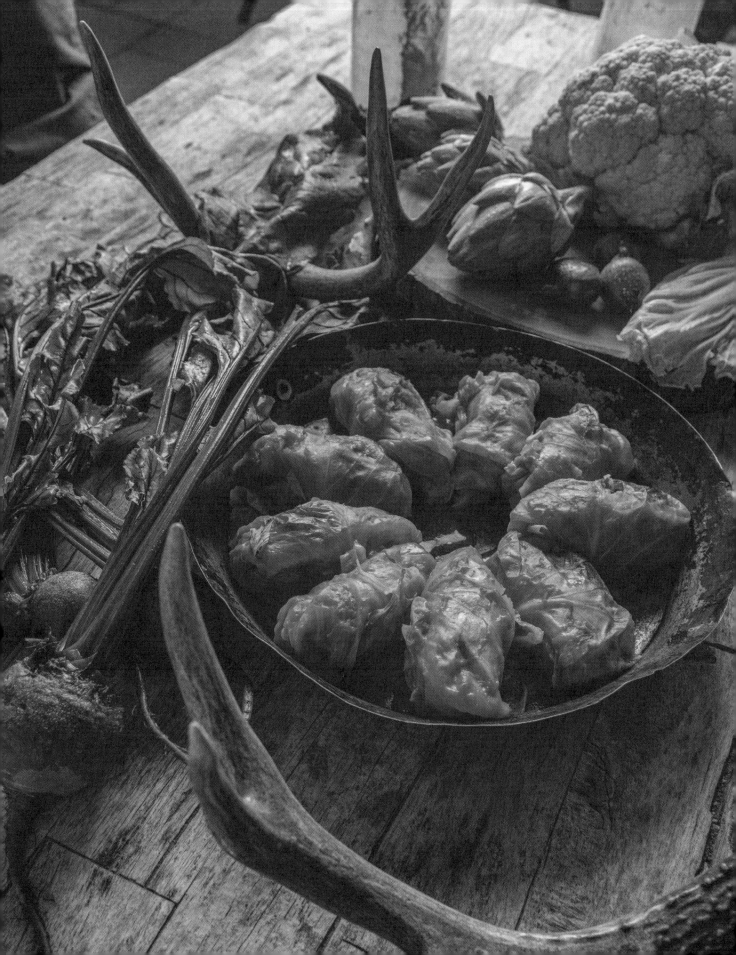

Thai Basil Ground Elk

SERVES 5

Chad Mendes's friend Rihana absolutely killed it with this recipe! Pun intended. This flavorful, Thai-inspired recipe may be our new favorite way to prepare ground meat. It's super easy to prepare and goes well over rice or mixed with pad Thai rice noodles. If Thai food is a favorite, we highly recommend this one!

2 tablespoons fish sauce

2 tablespoons soy sauce

2 tablespoons agave nectar

2 tablespoons Sriracha

2 tablespoons crushed red pepper

3 tablespoons toasted sesame oil, divided

2 garlic cloves, minced

1 shallot, sliced

1 large red bell pepper, seeded and sliced

1½ cups chopped Thai basil

2 pounds ground elk

Cooked white rice, to serve

In a small bowl, mix the fish sauce, soy sauce, agave, Sriracha, and crushed red pepper; set aside.

Heat 2 tablespoons of the sesame oil in a large frying pan over medium heat. Brown the garlic and shallot, then add the bell pepper and basil and cook for 3 minutes, or until the pepper is softened. Remove the pan from the heat.

In a separate frying pan, heat the remaining 1 tablespoon sesame oil over medium heat. Brown the elk, breaking it up with a spatula as it cooks, for 3–5 minutes. Add the sauce mixture and simmer until the elk is fully cooked, about 10 minutes more. Add the bell pepper mixture to the cooked meat and heat through. Serve over rice.

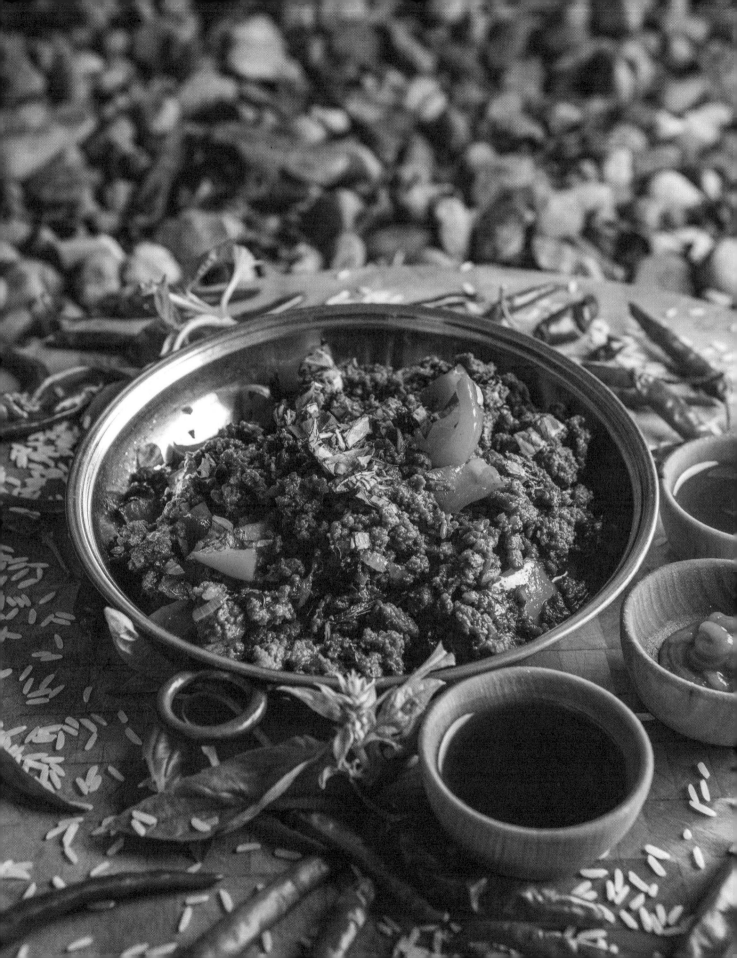

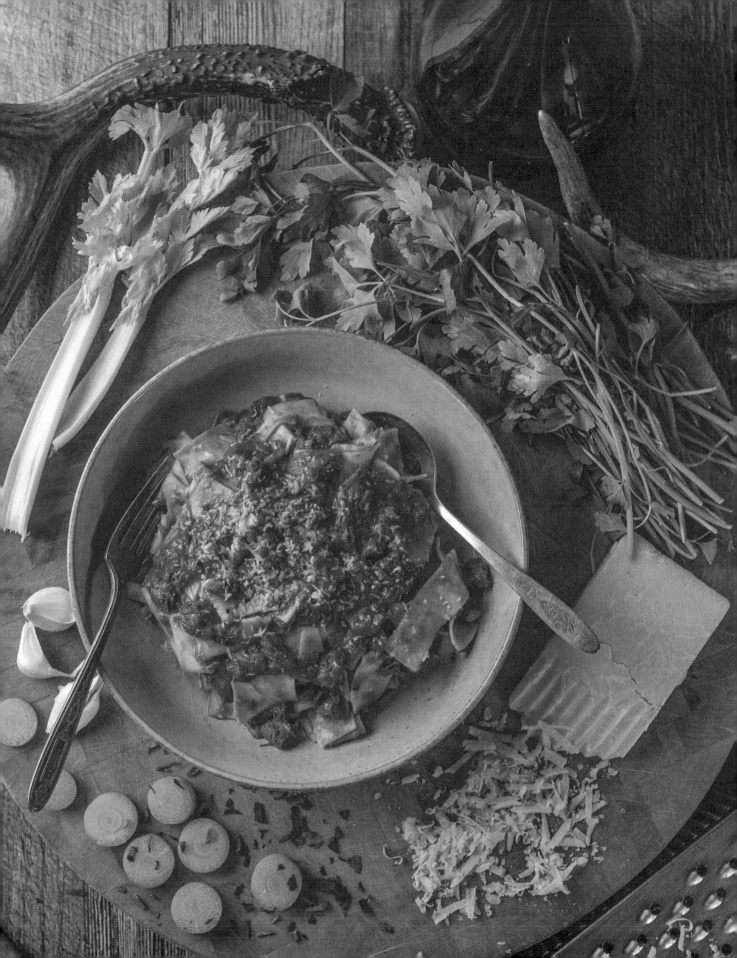

Slow-Cooked Venison Ragù

Chad Mendes has been on a huge cast-iron slow-cooking kick as of late. The amount of flavor created by cooking low and slow is just amazing. It lets you take cuts of meat that normally might be a little on the tougher side and break them down into super tender pieces. This stew pairs well with any red wine.

PASTA AND SAUCE

2–3 pounds venison roast, cut into 2-inch pieces

1 tablespoon salt, plus more to taste

Ground black pepper to taste

4 tablespoons olive oil, divided

1 sweet onion, diced

4 garlic cloves, minced

1 cup diced carrots

1 cup diced celery

1 (28-ounce) can diced fire-roasted tomatoes

3 tablespoons tomato paste

3 beef bouillon cubes

1 cup full-bodied red wine

2 cups water

4 thyme sprigs

3 bay leaves

1 pound dried egg pappardelle

TO SERVE

Grated parmesan cheese

Chopped fresh parsley

Season the venison cubes with the salt and several grinds of pepper.

In a large cast-iron pot or other heavy-bottomed pot, heat 1 tablespoon of the olive oil over high heat. Sear all sides of the venison pieces until very brown, working in batches if necessary. Transfer to a plate.

In the same pot, heat the remaining 3 tablespoons olive oil. Add the onion and cook until tender, 5–10 minutes. Add the garlic and cook for 2 minutes, or until fragrant, then add the carrots and celery. Sauté for 5 minutes, or until slightly softened. Add the fire-roasted tomatoes with their juice, tomato paste, bouillon cubes, red wine, water, thyme, and bay leaves to the pot. Return the venison to the pot, including any accumulated juices. Bring to a simmer, then reduce the heat until the sauce is at a very slow bubble. Cover and cook for 3–4 hours, until the venison is tender and falls apart easily.

continued

Once the venison is tender, use a potato masher or whisk to press and break apart the meat chunks into shreds in the sauce. Cover the pot again and simmer for another 30 minutes, or until the sauce is reduced and thickened. Remove and discard the thyme sprigs and bay leaves. Season with salt and pepper.

For the pasta, bring a large pot of water to a boil. Add the pappardelle and cook for 1 minute less than the recommended time on the package instructions. While the pasta is cooking, transfer 5 cups of the meat sauce to a large, deep frying pan or pot. Heat over high heat. When the pasta is ready, drain it, reserving ¾ cup of the cooking water. Add the pappardelle and reserved cooking water to the sauce and gently toss until the water has evaporated and the sauce has thickened. The sauce should coat and stick to the pasta. Plate the pasta, top with grated parmesan cheese and chopped parsley, and serve immediately.

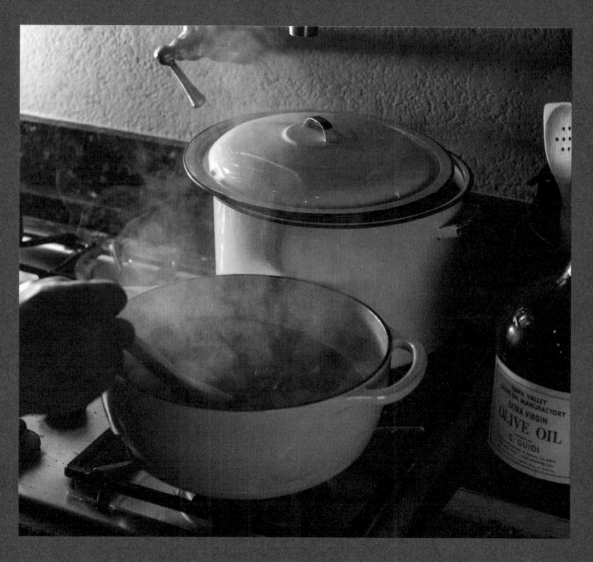

Korean BBQ Venison Street Tacos

SERVES 6

Tacos have always been a Mendes family favorite. We're always trying to find new and unique ways to create them, and this one definitely stands out! With a mix of both sweet and savory flavors, these tacos are sure to become a favorite.

VENISON

1 pound venison backstrap, thinly sliced

1 white onion, half sliced, half chopped, divided

3 green onions, 1 cut into 1-inch pieces, 2 thinly sliced, divided

½ pear, peeled, cored, and cut into chunks

3 garlic cloves, peeled and lightly smashed

⅓ cup soy sauce

3 tablespoons toasted sesame oil

3 tablespoons brown sugar

1 teaspoon ground black pepper

1 tablespoon neutral vegetable oil

1 teaspoon sesame seeds, for topping

SLAW

3 cups shredded green and/or red cabbage

¼ cup rice wine vinegar

1 tablespoon toasted sesame oil

Garlic powder to taste

Salt and ground black pepper to taste

AVOCADO MASH

2 avocados, peeled and pitted

Garlic powder to taste

Pinch sesame seeds

Salt and ground black pepper to taste

TO SERVE

Small corn or flour tortillas

Put the venison and sliced white onion in a large bowl.

In a blender, blend the chopped white onion, big green onion pieces, pear, garlic cloves, soy sauce, sesame oil, brown sugar, and pepper until smooth. Pour the mixture over the venison and onion slices and toss to combine. Cover and refrigerate for 30 minutes.

While the meat marinates, make the slaw and avocado mash. In a large bowl, combine the cabbage, rice wine vinegar, sesame oil, garlic powder, and salt and pepper. Toss to combine. In a separate bowl, mash the avocados with garlic powder, sesame seeds, and salt and pepper. Cover and refrigerate both until ready to serve.

continued

In a large cast-iron skillet, heat the vegetable oil over medium-high heat. Remove the venison and onion slices from the marinade and pat dry. Cook the venison and onion, stirring occasionally, until browned. Transfer to a serving dish and top with the sesame seeds and thinly sliced green onion.

Wipe out the skillet and return it to the heat. Heat the tortillas for about 45 seconds on each side. To make the tacos, layer the meat on each tortilla and top with avocado mash and slaw.

Chad Mendes says: "Starting with cold or partially frozen meat will make slicing easier."

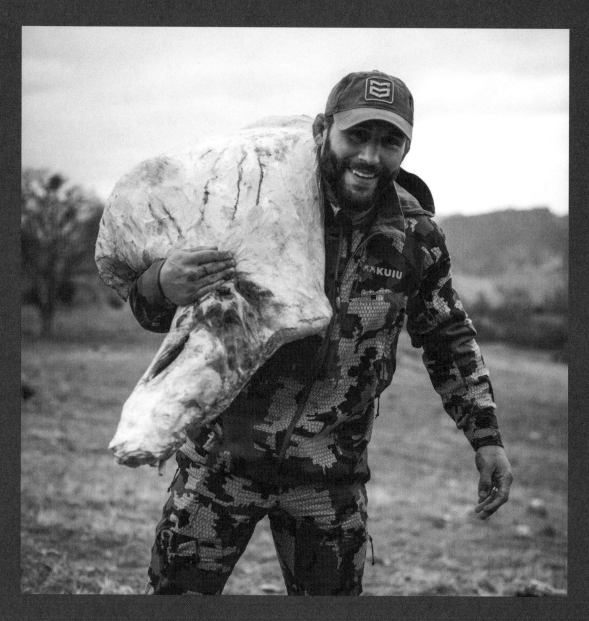

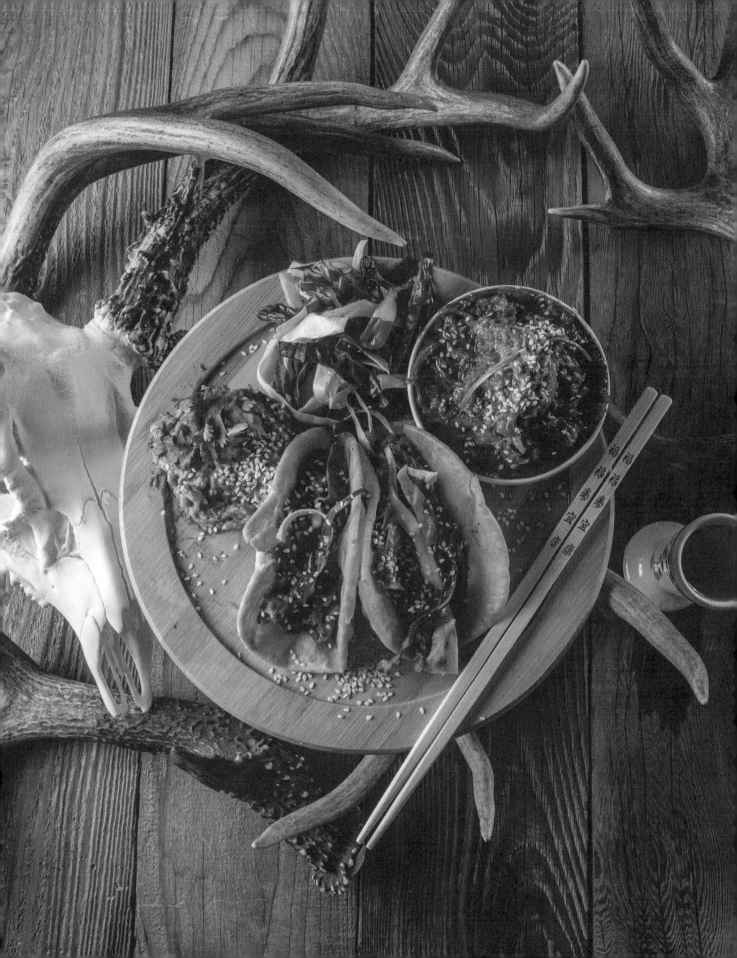

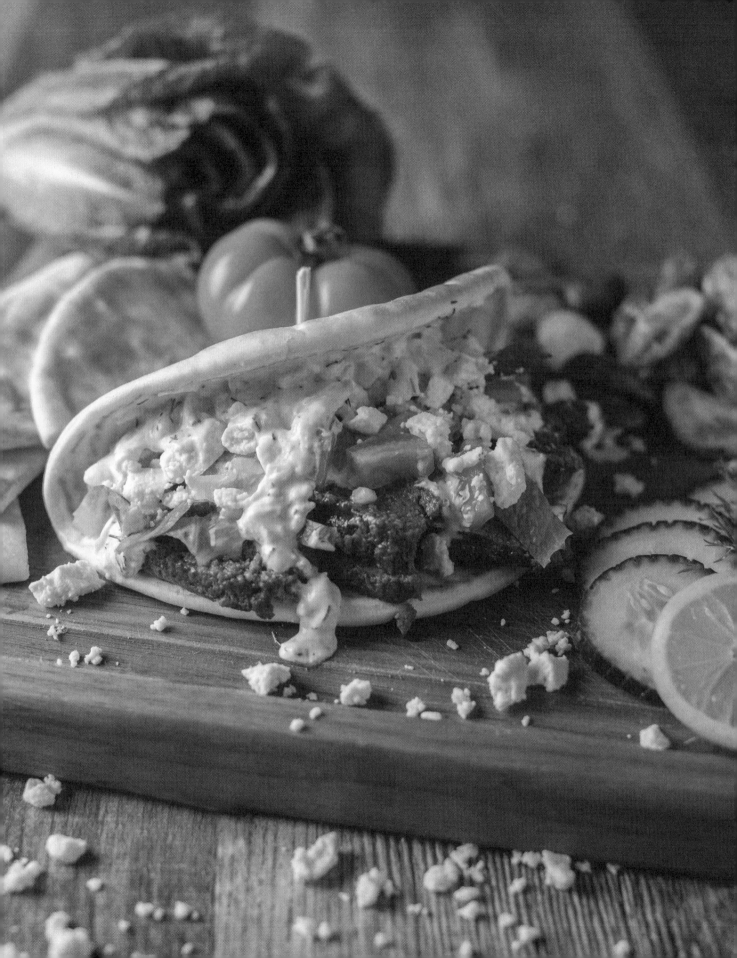

Elk Gyros

MAKES 4 GYROS

Chad Mendes was introduced to Greek food right after college. "I moved up to Sacramento with my teammate and friend Urijah Faber," he says. "He took me to a local Greek restaurant after practice one day and told me I had to try these gyros. I gave it a shot and have been hooked on them ever since. I love the unique flavor that elk, wild boar, or even whitetail adds to this recipe."

TZATZIKI

2 cups grated cucumber

1½ cups plain Greek yogurt

2 tablespoons olive oil

1 tablespoon lemon juice

1 garlic clove, minced

2 tablespoons chopped fresh dill

½ teaspoon salt

ELK

1 pound ground elk (straight grind or fat added)

¼ cup finely chopped fresh mint

1 garlic clove, minced

1 large egg yolk

1 tablespoon ground black pepper

2½ teaspoons salt

GYROS

4 pita breads

1 cup chopped lettuce

1 tomato, chopped

½ cup chopped white onion

½ cup crumbled feta cheese

Preheat your grill (we use a Traeger) to 450°F. Have ready four metal skewers.

To make the tzatziki, press or squeeze the excess moisture from the grated cucumber and put the cucumber in a large bowl. Add the Greek yogurt, olive oil, lemon juice, garlic, dill, and salt and mix well. Cover and chill for 15 minutes to let the flavors blend.

In a large bowl, combine the ground elk, mint, garlic, egg yolk, pepper, and salt and mix well. Form the mixture into four logs, each about 5 inches long. Insert a skewer from the bottom all the way through the top of each log. Place the meat skewers directly on the grill grate. Cook for about 3 minutes on each side, until cooked through. Transfer the skewers to a platter.

Place the pita breads on the grill and cook until warm and soft, 1–2 minutes.

Spread some tzatziki on the inside of each pita. Remove the meat from the skewers and place in the pitas. Top with lettuce, tomato, onion, and feta.

Backcountry Elk Hunt

Chad Mendes

A trip to northern Oregon was my first experience hunting elk on public lands outside of Utah. Abby (then my fiancée), my dad, and I decided to find a drop camp outfitter to pack all our stuff into the backcountry. We met with the outfitter two days before we were set to head in. They loaded up all our gear on horses and packed it all into a solid area we would call home for the week. The next day, the three of us hopped on our mountain bikes and set off for the 5-mile trek in.

After close to three hours of riding, we started to get a little worried we had missed a turn somewhere. We ended up running into someone and quickly found out that the outfitter had given us the wrong directions—we had been riding the wrong way the entire time! It was a long, grueling day to say the least, but we did finally end up making it to our camp. Completely worn out, we decided to lie down for a nap after getting all our stuff set up.

We woke to a light rain hitting the canvas tent walls. As I peeked my head outside, I noticed a beautiful bull elk feeding in the meadow about 150 yards in front of us! I quickly grabbed my camera and started filming. The season opened in the morning, and we were extremely hopeful that we might see this guy again.

With multiple close calls the next few days on that bull and a few others, we decided it was time to head down into the big canyons. After about a 6-mile hike down into the breaks, we finally found a bull. With Abby sneaking along behind me with camera in hand, we closed the distance to inside 100 yards. The only problem was we lost sight of him. Knowing he was most likely very close, we slowed everything way, way down. As we reached the base of a hill inside the dense timber, I handed Abby my shooting sticks and told her to wait there as I crept up to peek over. I had made it about 20 yards up the hill when a loud *crash* echoed behind me! I crouched down and looked back, only to see Abby almost in tears. She had bent down to try to film me through the trees and lost hold of the shooting sticks.

Without knowing exactly where the bull was (but knowing that he had most likely heard the noise), I sat for a few minutes to let things calm down and listen to see if I could hear any footsteps. With nothing happening,

I started creeping back up to the top. As my view started to crest over, I immediately caught a glimpse of his ivory antler tips 50 yards in front of me! I could tell from the way they were facing he was looking right in my direction. With my rifle loaded, I waited for the antler tips to turn so I could make my move. After what seemed like hours, he finally turned his head to the right and I quickly raised up and found his shoulder in my crosshairs. With one perfectly placed bullet, we had just harvested enough meat to feed our entire wedding party just a few months away!

Now, at this time in our relationship, Abby had never seen a big game animal harvested and had definitely never been a part of breaking one down in the field. With about 30 minutes of light left, we knew we had a lot of work ahead of us. With nothing for light but our head-lamps, Abby and I broke down that entire bull ourselves. We hung all four quarters up in a big tree and loaded up as much meat as we could. We began our pack-out around 8:30 p.m. Being in wolf, bear, and mountain lion country made us very uneasy, especially carrying a bunch of meat on our backs and having only two dimming lights to lead the way. To this day, the pack-out of that canyon was one of the most physically and mentally challenging things we have ever been through together. We didn't end up getting back to camp and meeting back up with my dad till around 10:30 p.m., but man was it worth it all!

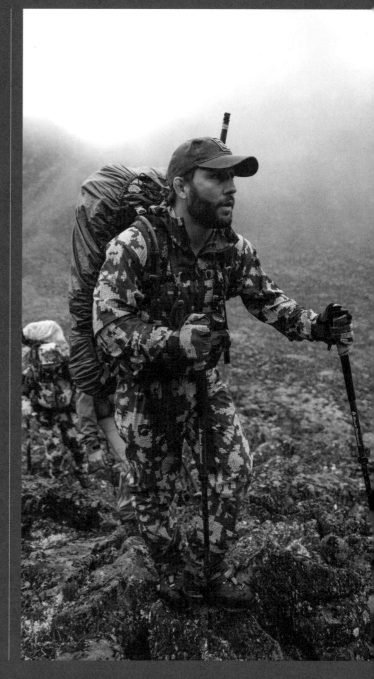

BBJ's Famous Biscuits and Gravy

SERVES 4

Biscuits and sausage gravy is what Chad Mendes's mother in-law, Momma Judy, makes every time we visit. It's packed with so much flavor that Chad can't help but go back for seconds—sometimes even thirds!

---

1 (16-ounce) can refrigerated buttermilk biscuits

1 pound bulk wild boar breakfast sausage or any breakfast sausage

3 tablespoons chopped yellow onion

1 teaspoon ground sage

Garlic powder to taste

Seasoned salt (such as Lawry's) to taste

Ground black pepper to taste

1 cup all-purpose flour

4 cups whole milk, divided

Bake the biscuits according to the package instructions.

Heat a large frying pan over medium heat. Add the sausage, onion, and all the seasonings and cook, breaking up the sausage with a spatula, until the meat is done and the onion is soft, about 8 minutes.

In a separate bowl, whisk the flour and 3 cups of the milk until smooth.

Turn the heat down to low and slowly pour the flour and milk mixture over the meat. Cook, stirring constantly. As the mixture thickens, slowly add the remaining 1 cup milk into the gravy and cook until it reaches the desired consistency. Divide the biscuits between plates or bowls and ladle the sausage gravy on top.

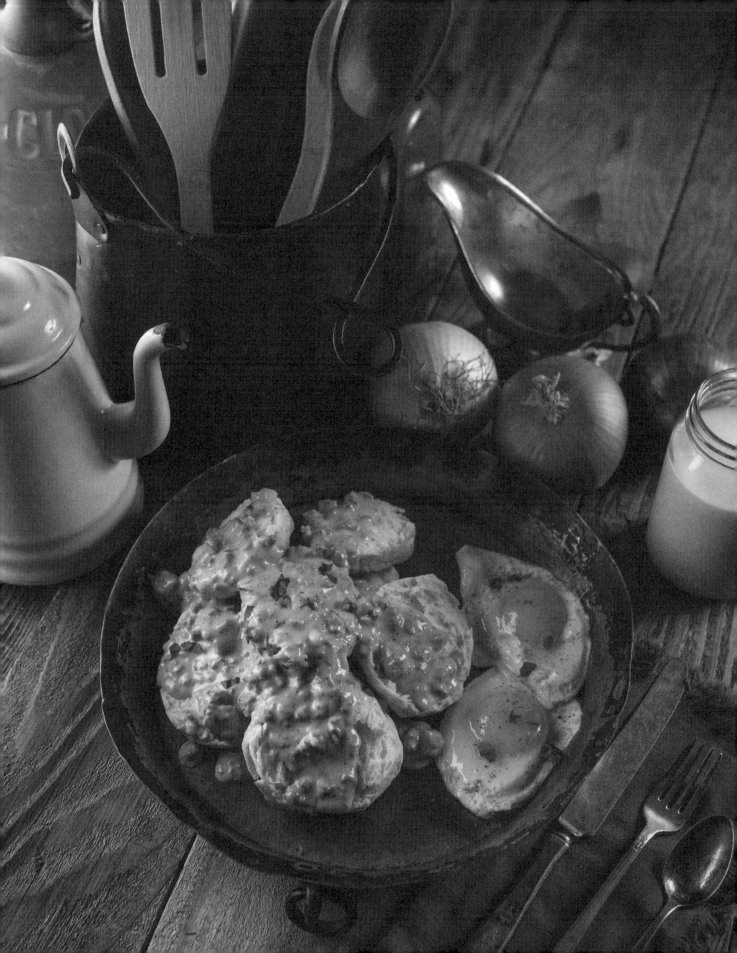

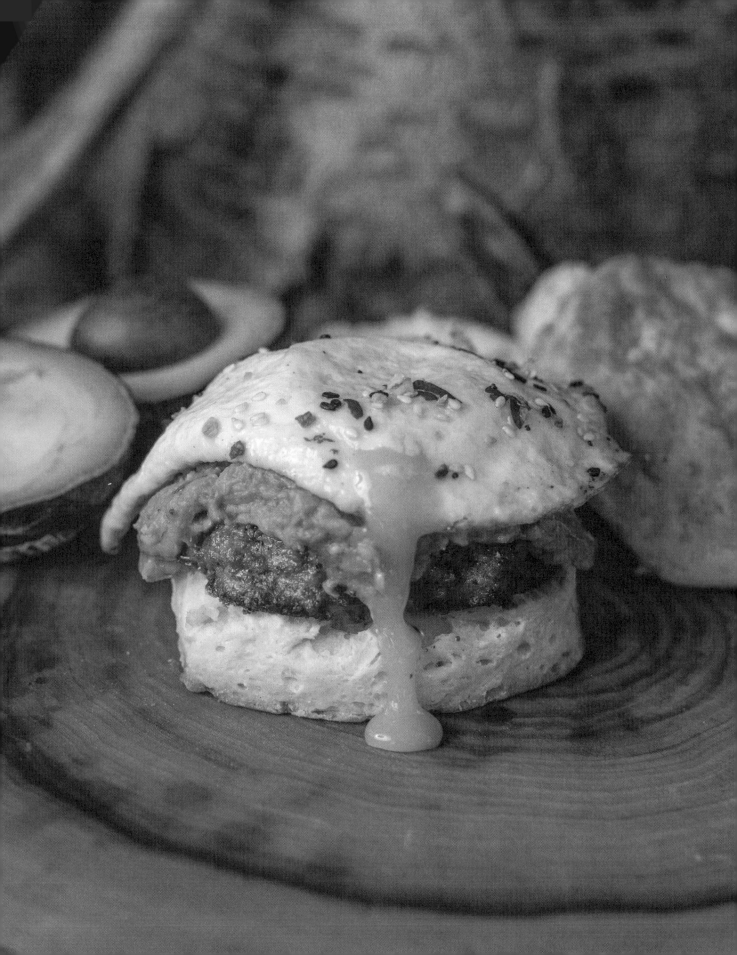

The Money Breakfast Sandwich

SERVES 2

Chad Mendes's wife, Abby, might love this breakfast recipe even more than he does. You could take things to the next level by using a homemade buttermilk biscuit (as pictured) instead of the English muffin and 6-minute soft-boiled eggs instead of fried. It takes a bit longer but is an amazing addition to an already delicious breakfast!

---

1 regular or whole wheat English muffin

1 tablespoon unsalted butter

½ avocado, peeled and pitted

Pinch garlic powder

Salt to taste

4 ounces bulk venison breakfast sausage

1 tablespoon black truffle oil

1 lemon wedge

2 large eggs

Cooking spray

1 tablespoon microgreens

2 pinches everything bagel seasoning

Separate the English muffin and toast both sides. When done, spread butter on each half.

In a small bowl, mash the avocado with the garlic powder and salt.

Form the venison breakfast sausage into two thin patties about the same size around as the English muffin halves.

Heat a medium frying pan over medium heat. Cook the sausage patties until cooked through, 3–4 minutes per side. Place one on top of each English muffin half. Add a generous scoop of avocado mash on top of each patty. Drizzle a bit of the truffle oil over the avocado mash, along with a squeeze of lemon.

Spray the same frying pan with cooking spray and cook the eggs to the desired doneness (Mendes likes his over medium). Add them to the top of the avocado mash. Garnish with a bit of micro-greens and top with a pinch of the everything bagel seasoning.

Wild Boar and Feta Cheese Stuffed Mushrooms

SERVES 4

Chad Mendes says, "This is a great recipe for anyone looking to cut back on starchy carbs but still wanting something absolutely delicious! This was one of my favorite recipes to make during my fight camps when I was losing weight." The firm, almost nutty flavor of the mushrooms pairs beautifully with the wild boar sausage, feta, pine nuts, and balsamic.

---

4 large portobello mushrooms

1 tablespoon olive oil, plus more for drizzling

½ white onion, chopped

2 garlic cloves, minced

1 pound bulk wild boar Italian sausage

2 cups chopped spinach

¼ cup pine nuts

¼ cup feta cheese

Balsamic vinegar

Salt to taste (optional)

Preheat your grill (we use a Traeger) or oven to 400°F.

To prep the mushrooms, first remove the stems. With a spoon, gently scrape out all the gills from the underside. With a damp paper towel, wipe away any excess dirt from the caps.

Heat the olive oil in a large frying pan over medium-high heat. Sauté the onion until tender, 5–10 minutes. Add the garlic and cook for 2 minutes, or until fragrant. Push the onion and garlic to the edges of the pan. Add the sausage to the center of the pan and cook, breaking up the meat with a spatula, until cooked through, 6–8 minutes. About halfway through, start mixing the onion and garlic into the meat. Add the spinach, pine nuts, and feta cheese and stir to combine. When the spinach is wilted, remove the pan from the heat.

Pile some of the mixture into the gilled side of each mushroom cap. Drizzle a bit of olive oil and balsamic over the top. The sausage should have plenty of salt, but if not, you can add a few pinches now. Set the mushrooms on the grill (or on a rimmed baking sheet if using the oven) and cook until tender, 15–20 minutes.

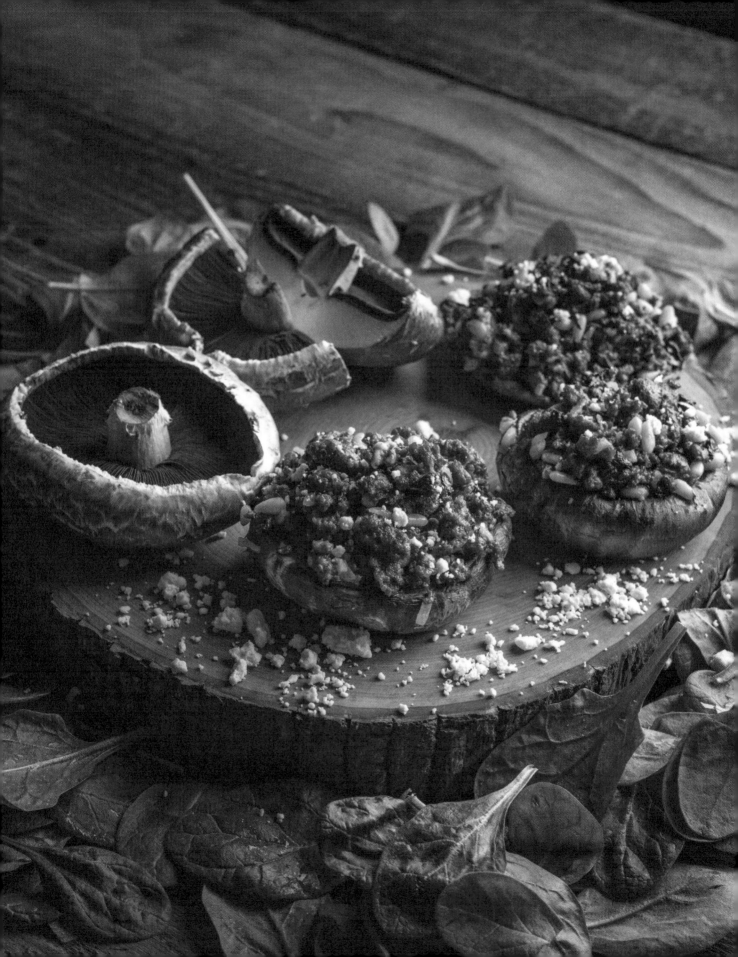

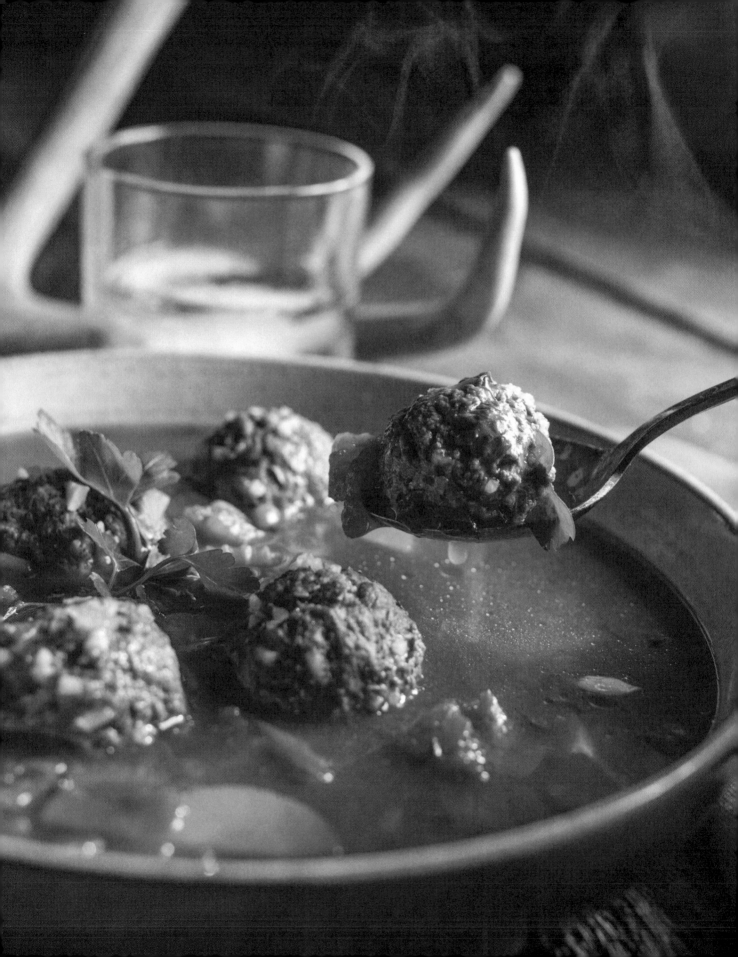

Axis Deer Meatball Soup

SERVES 8

This recipe features a wild game twist to one of Chad Mendes's favorite Mexican soups: "With so many south-of-the-border flavors and one of my all-time favorite wild game meats added to the mix, this soup is a tough one to beat on a cold day!"

---

3 tablespoons olive oil

1 large sweet onion, chopped

2 garlic cloves, minced

2 quarts beef stock

1 quart water

½ cup tomato sauce

1 (14.5-ounce) can diced fire-roasted
  tomatoes

2 large carrots, peeled and sliced

2 celery ribs, sliced

1 pound ground axis deer with beef fat added

⅓ cup uncooked white rice

¼ cup (loosely packed) chopped fresh
  spearmint

¼ cup (loosely packed) chopped fresh parsley

1 large egg

2 teaspoons salt

1 teaspoon ground black pepper

2 cups frozen or fresh peas

1 teaspoon chopped fresh oregano

½ teaspoon cayenne pepper

½ cup chopped fresh cilantro, for garnish

In a large pot, heat the olive oil over medium-high heat. Sauté the onion until tender, about 5 minutes. Add the garlic and cook for another minute, until fragrant. Add the beef stock, water, tomato sauce, and fire-roasted tomatoes with their juice. Bring to a boil, then reduce the heat to a simmer. Add the carrots and celery.

Meanwhile, in a large bowl, combine the deer meat, rice, mint, parsley, egg, salt, and black pepper. Form the mixture into meatballs about 1 inch in diameter. Add the meatballs to the simmering soup, one at a time, taking care not to break them. Cover and simmer for 30 minutes.

Add the peas, oregano, and cayenne toward the end of the cooking time and stir to combine. Let simmer for a few minutes, until the peas are heated through. Ladle into bowls and garnish with the cilantro.

Italian Wedding Soup with Elk Meatballs

SERVES 8

We have been preparing this traditional recipe for years and finally get to bring it to the public. Through trial and error, we have achieved the perfectly seasoned wild game version of a classic. Get your spoons ready!

ELK MEATBALLS

1 pound bulk elk sausage (any flavor)

2 slices white bread, finely crumbled

¼ cup chopped fresh parsley

1 sprig oregano, leaves chopped

½ cup grated parmesan cheese

1 large egg

½ teaspoon salt

¼ teaspoon ground black pepper

1 tablespoon olive oil

SOUP

1 tablespoon olive oil

1 medium yellow onion, diced

1 large carrot, peeled and finely diced

2 celery ribs, finely diced

3 garlic gloves, minced

8 cups chicken stock

1 cup uncooked acini or other small pasta

1 cup chopped baby spinach, escarole, or kale

Salt and ground black pepper to taste

Grated parmesan cheese, for garnish

Combine all the meatball ingredients except the olive oil in a large bowl. Knead everything together with your hands, then pinch off small pieces and roll into bite-size balls.

In a large skillet, heat the olive oil over medium-high heat. Add as many meatballs to the pan as will fit without touching, and cook for 4–5 minutes, flipping halfway through. Transfer the cooked meatballs to a plate. Cook the remaining meatballs.

In a large soup pot, heat the olive oil over medium-high heat. Sauté the onion, carrot, and celery until tender. Stir in the garlic and cook for 30 seconds. Add the chicken stock and bring to a boil. Add the pasta and meatballs. Reduce the heat to medium, cover, and cook until the pasta is done, 10–12 minutes.

Stir in the spinach and cook until it wilts, then season with salt and pepper. Serve with parmesan cheese for topping.

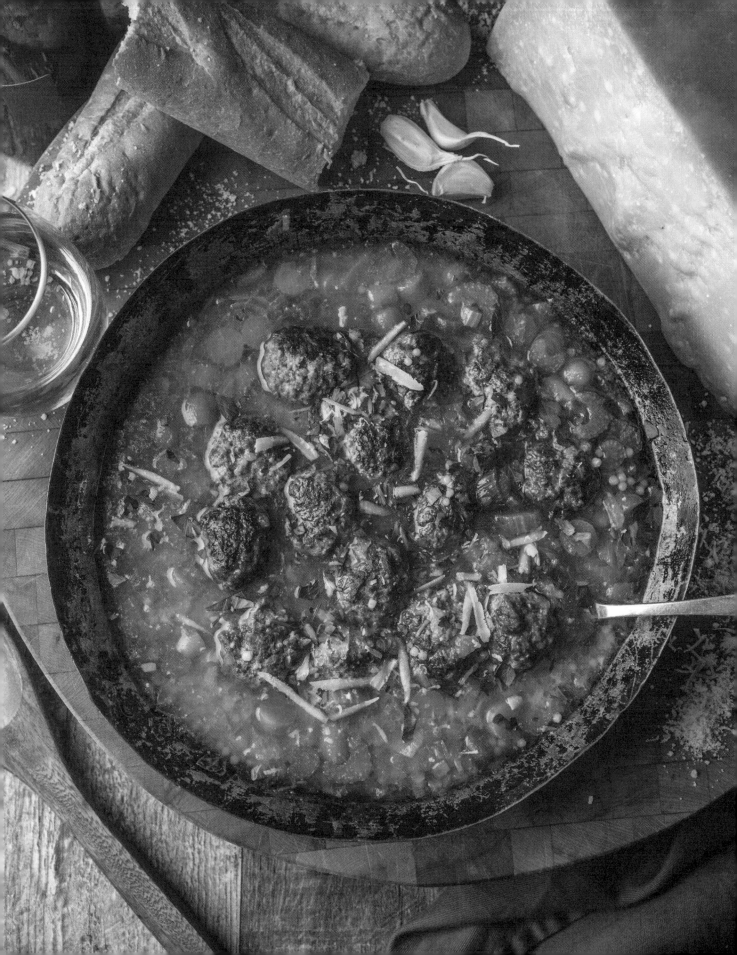

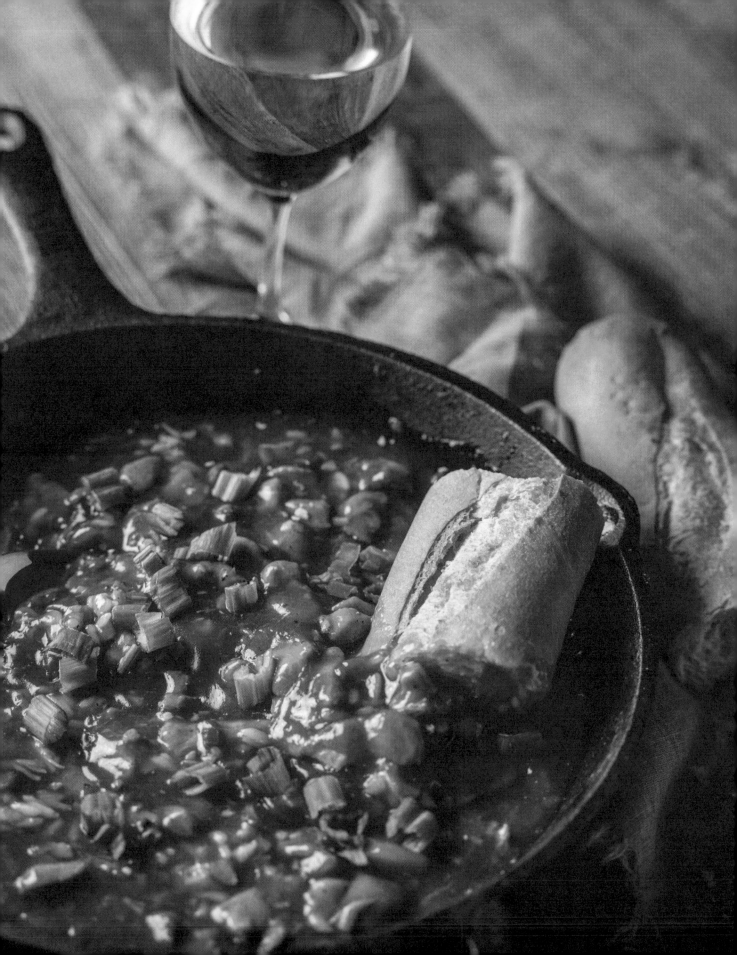

Squirrel Stew

There is nothing like being with a group of Cajuns in hunting camp and having them teach you about their culture. Our friend Miss Chelly Cross is one of those who holds nothing back when it comes to her passion for cooking. To be in her kitchen is to be at the epicenter of culinary flair! She hunts squirrels, and this recipe is her go-to for cooking at duck camp. We are so happy we get to share it with you. Obviously, squirrels aren't exactly big game, but they're delicious and a great food source. Bushytails are fast, and they can scale a tree in seconds, so you will have to be on your A game to get them into the pot!

½ cup neutral vegetable oil

6 squirrels, skinned and cut into serving pieces

2 yellow onions, diced

1 green bell pepper, seeded and diced

4 garlic cloves, minced

2 packages onion soup mix

3 packages brown gravy mix

2 tablespoons Cajun seasoning, such as Tony Chachere's

4–6 cups water

Heat the vegetable oil in a large Dutch oven or cast-iron pot over medium-high heat. Fry the squirrel pieces until brown, 3–4 minutes per side. Transfer to a plate.

Add the onions, bell pepper, and garlic to the pot and cook for 5 minutes, or until the onions become soft and translucent. Return the squirrel pieces to the pot, along with the soup mix, gravy mix, and Cajun seasoning. Add enough water to cover the squirrel pieces. Bring to a boil and simmer for 1 hour, or until tender. Ladle into shallow bowls and serve.

Now the Real Work Begins: Field Dressing Deer

Once the adrenaline has worn off, the photos have been taken, and you have placed the tag on your deer, the real work begins. I prefer the "gutless" method when field dressing deer. This technique works for most big game animals as well.

First decide whether or not you are mounting the deer you have harvested. If you are, start by skinning the area typically used for a shoulder mount. (Obviously if you are doing a full-body mount, the entire animal will need to be skinned.) For your typical shoulder mount, start by making an entrance in the hide at the base of the skull in line with the spine. Cut down the spine to about mid-belly; it is better to have more hide when dropping off your deer at the taxidermist. Then cut around the belly until you meet up with the original cut on the spine. At this point, skin all the way up to the head, tubing and removing the lower front leg hide. Tubing the legs can be tricky—you want to remove the leg at the middle joint and peel the hide down off the shoulder without cutting the hide around the leg. The hide on the leg will come off in one piece like a tube. Once the neck is exposed, remove the head and cape as close to the base of the skull as possible. This leaves you with the head, cape, and horns all together. I choose to leave the delicate facial caping to the taxidermist whenever possible. Your trophy is preserved. Now for the meat!

Time is of the essence when breaking down your game, but it is important to be careful while using knives not only to protect yourself, but also to keep your meat in good condition. I start by skinning down the rest of the deer. Once skinned, remove the backstraps on either side of the spine. This is choice meat, so do it carefully. Running a knife down the side of the spine as close to the bone as possible frees the meat from spine. Cut down toward the ribs, removing the large sections of meat whole. Now remove the front legs whole. These are floating limbs, meaning they have no ball-and-socket joint to deal with. Cut around the large shoulder muscle and down under the armpit area; lifting upward will help determine where to cut. The front legs will come off whole, ready for the game bag.

Now on to the back legs, which are a little more difficult. The back legs are jointed to the pelvis area with a ball-and-socket joint. With the animal on its side, lift the leg upward and start to cut the around the large muscle group at the top of the leg, starting near the belly and cutting around. Pay close attention to the internal organs, as they will be all around the area you are working in. Cut in until you find the ball joint; moving the leg up and down will help determine where the joint is located. Once all the meat is cut, you will be able to dislocate the joint with a sharp lift upward. There is a lot of meat here, so take your time and make good cuts.

Ready for the crown jewels? The tenderloins can be retrieved by making a cut below the last rib bone large enough to fit your hand inside. The internal organs will be up against these tenderloins, so you need to be careful when cutting them off the animal. Place your hand in the cut and feel up under the spine area, and you will feel these two muscles running parallel with the spine on either side, like a smaller backstrap, but lower on the animal. Once you locate them, carefully cut them out, being mindful of the internal organs.

Finishing up the process comes down to many factors, so check your local regulations for wanton waste laws. If the temperatures are cool, you have room in your pack, or you just want to get all the meat you can, now is the time. The neck can be deboned as well as the ribs. Once you have done this, you should have all your fresh venison ready to be butchered.

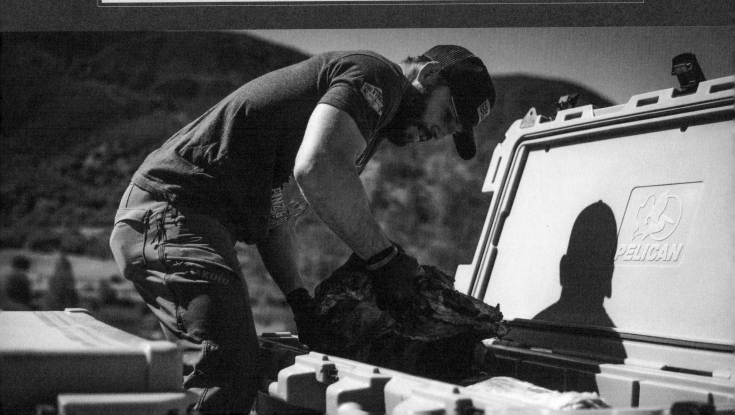

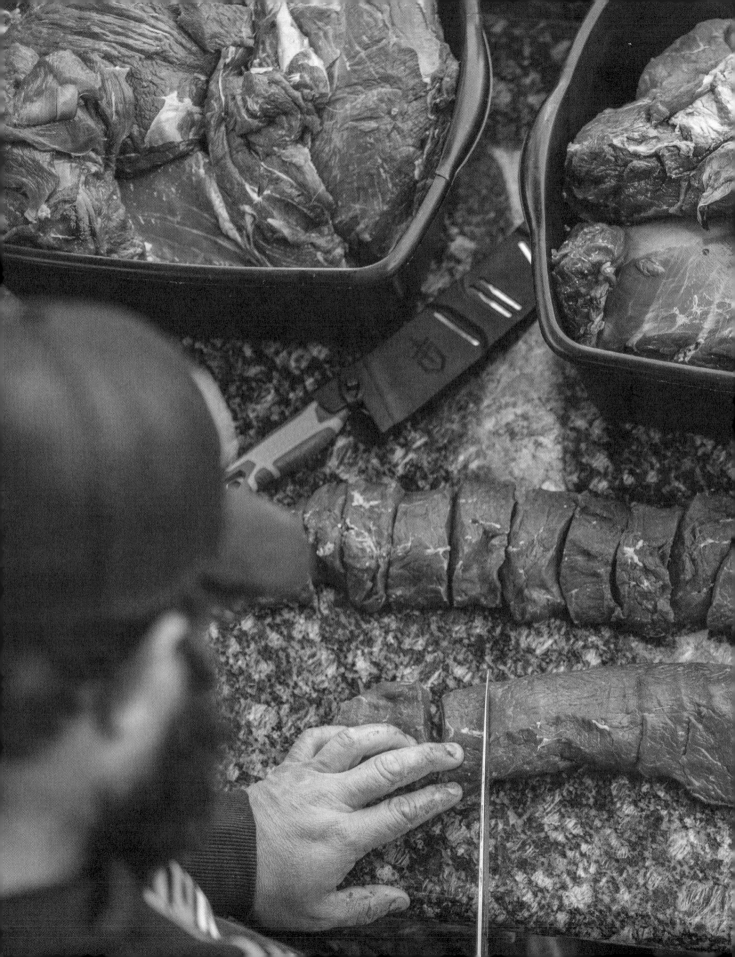

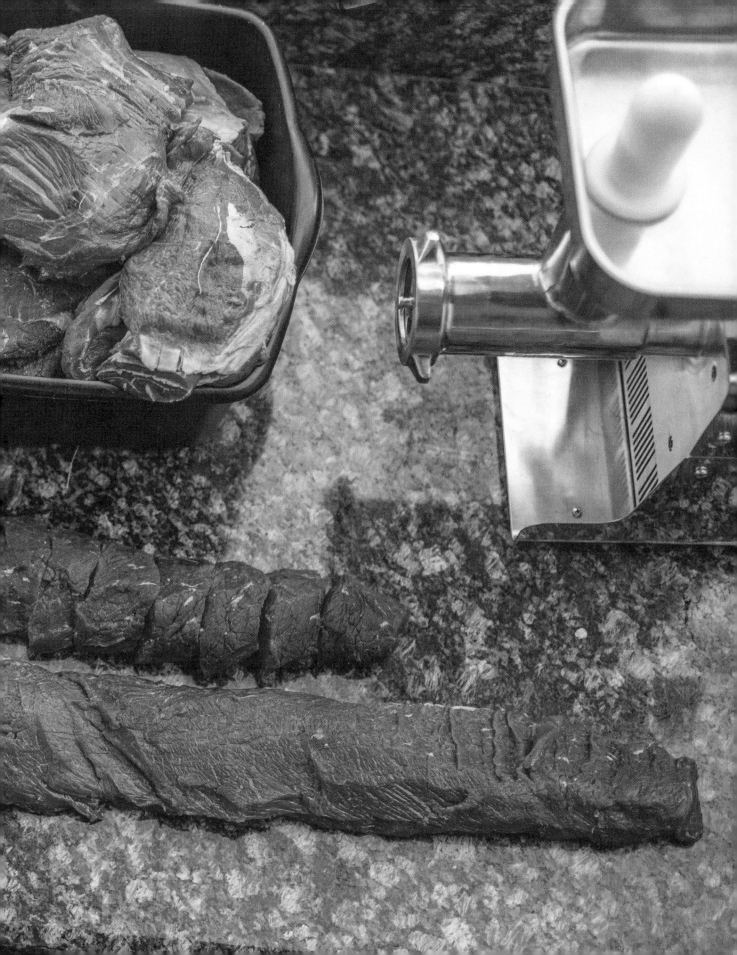

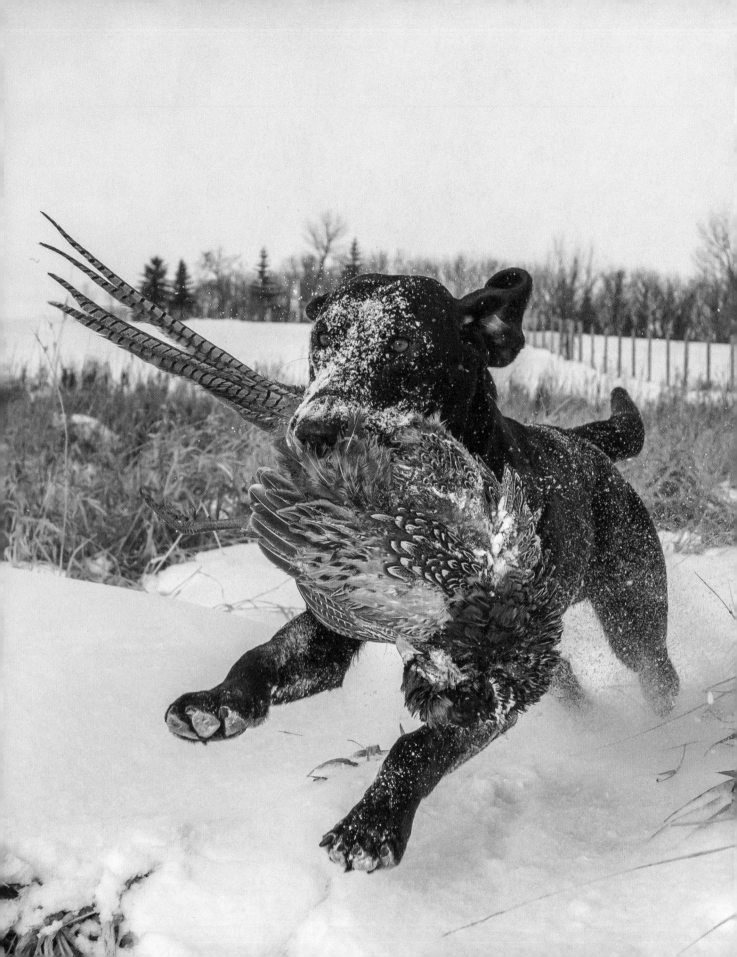

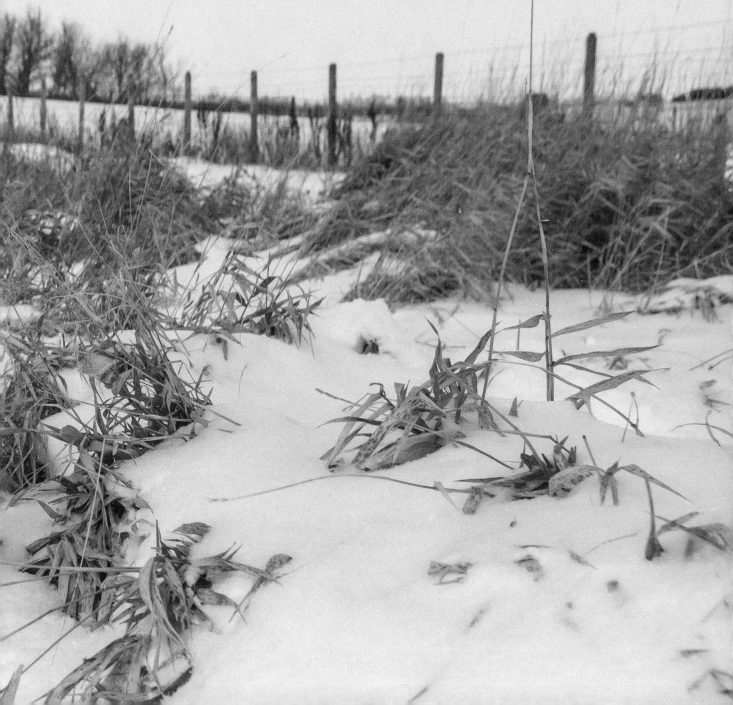

UPLAND
GAME BIRDS

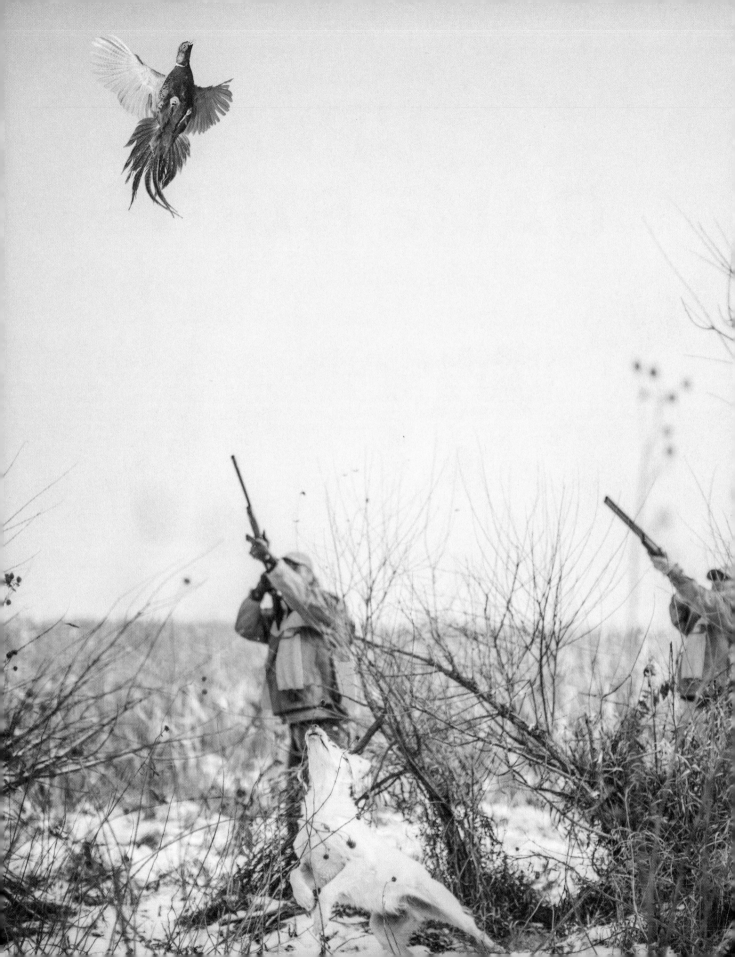

When it comes to upland bird hunting, there are two points that we have to make: the point that it tastes amazing and the point of the pointers! Upland bird dogs are referred to as pointers for good reason. Their noses are down as they scour the terrain in search of a quail or pheasant or chukar partridge. When they establish the scent pattern of a covey of birds, they become like a statue with their nose to the ground and their tail straight up in the air . . . on point! This is when an upland hunter is at their all-time high. The sight of a Brittany spaniel or English pointer working an area is hard to equal in the world of hunting! And it all comes full circle after the shot is fired and the bird busts up in the air. That same dog retrieves the bird, delivers it to hand, and watches as the hunter carefully places the bird into the back pocket of their vest.

Now it's time to get creative. Believe us when we say you can get creative with your upland game bird dishes using wild turkey, quail, and chukar. We have put together a variety of recipes for you and will leave it up to you to which one to try first. Now watch for that point!

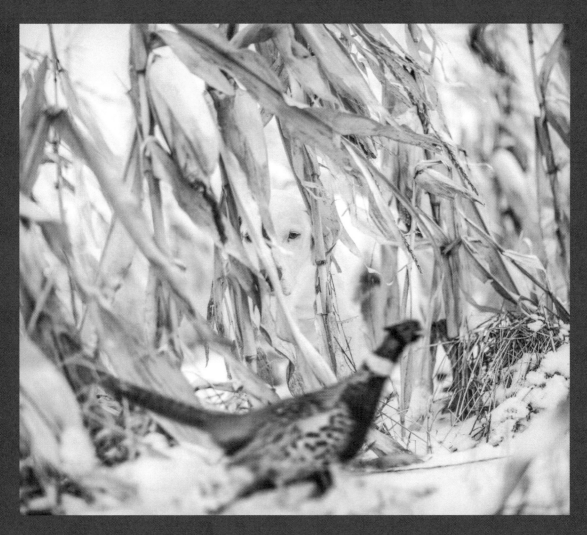

Mossy Pond's Smother-Fried Quail

SERVES 6-8

Mossy Pond Retrievers, located in southern Georgia, is known for training and turning out the best darn hunting dogs in the country! These dogs will fetch a duck, run you up a pheasant, and point you up a quail. When owners Brad and Ellen Arington prepare this dish, they wow every person sitting at their big table. Quail are quick and they fly fast, but not as fast as this dish will disappear from your plate!

---

2 quarts buttermilk

¾ cup hot sauce (Brad and Ellen like Texas Pete)

10 quail, dressed and rinsed

Neutral vegetable oil, for frying

1 teaspoon MSG

Salt and ground black pepper to taste

2¼ cups all-purpose flour, divided

4–6 tablespoons seasoned salt (such as Lawry's)

4 onions, sliced

3–4 cups water

In a large bowl, combine the buttermilk and hot sauce. Add the quail and turn to coat. Cover and let them marinate in the refrigerator for 24 hours.

Pour a few inches of vegetable oil into a large, heavy-bottomed pot (enough so that the quail will be submerged when you add them). Heat over medium-high heat until the oil is simmering.

While the oil is heating, drain the quail and season well with the MSG, salt, and pepper.

Combine 2 cups of the flour and the seasoned salt in a large bowl. Roll the quail in the flour mixture until it is well coated. Shake off the excess flour and carefully drop the quail into the hot oil. Work in batches as necessary to not crowd the pot.

Fry until the quail are golden brown, 6–8 minutes. Lift them from the pot with tongs and let them drain on a wire rack.

When all the quail are done, carefully pour off all but ¼ cup oil from the pot. Add the sliced onions and cook, stirring frequently, until golden brown.

Stir in the remaining ¼ cup flour and cook, stirring constantly, until the flour browns. Slowly stir in the water until you reach the desired consistency and thickness for your gravy. Once the gravy begins to boil, turn the heat down to low. Return the quail to the pot and let them simmer in the gravy for 20–25 minutes, then serve.

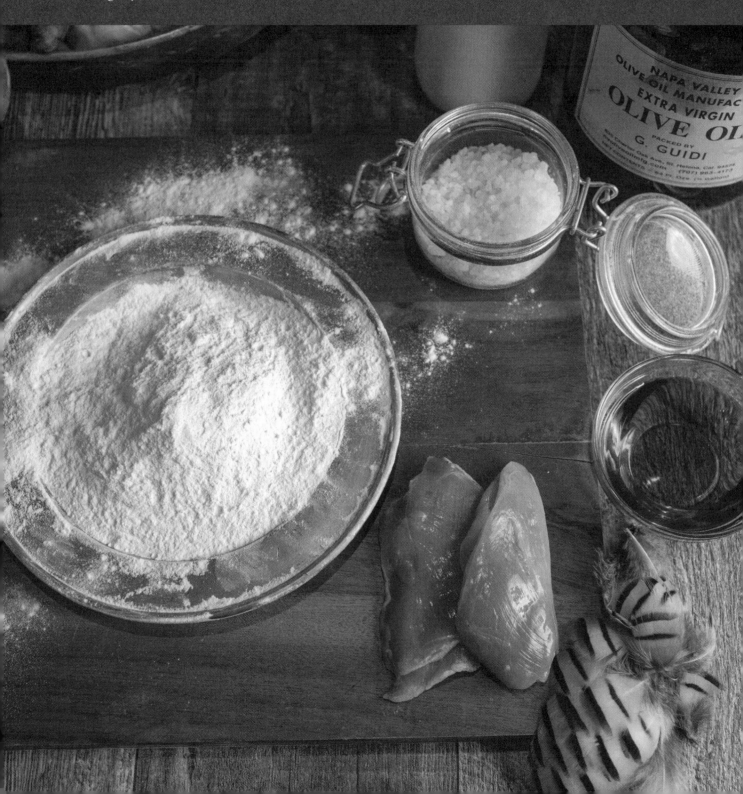

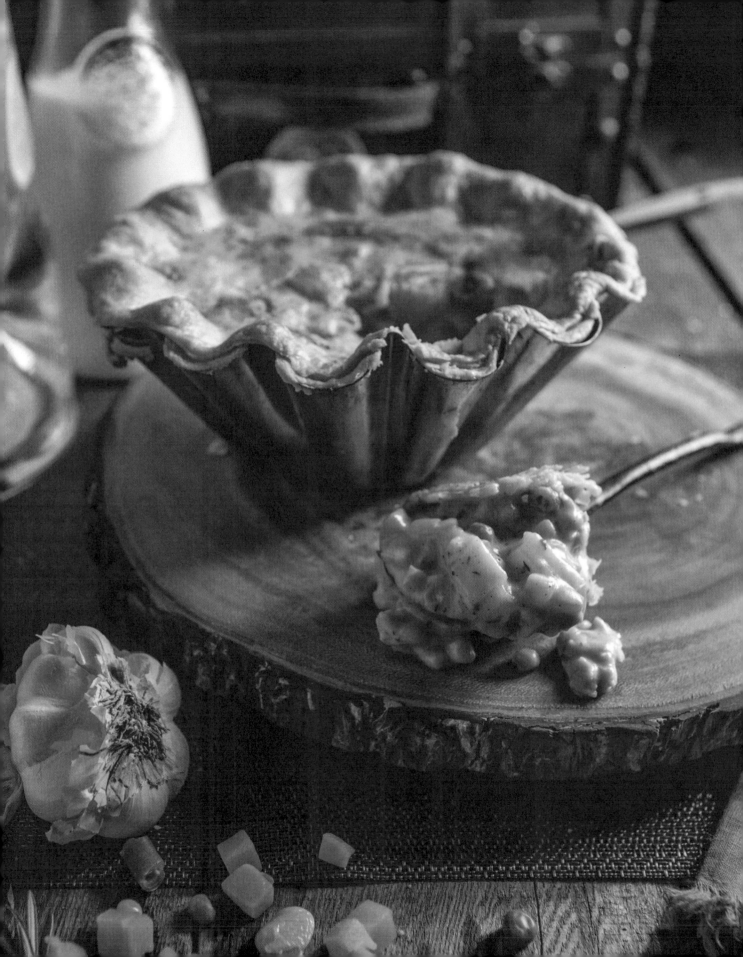

Wild Turkey Pot Pie

SERVES 4

This is one of our favorite hearty comfort food meals and will keep you full for hours. The creamy, savory filling topped with flaky crust will become one of your go-to's with wild turkey! If it's a mature bird, half a breast will get you the amount of turkey you need. For a young jake or hen, use the full breast.

⅓ cup unsalted butter

1 white onion, diced

½ wild turkey breast, cut into bite-size pieces (about 2 pounds)

⅓ cup all-purpose flour

1½ teaspoons The Provider Covey Rub or your favorite spice rub

1½ teaspoons ground black pepper

¼ teaspoon chopped fresh thyme

¼ teaspoon chopped fresh rosemary

1 cup chicken stock

⅔ cup milk or plain unsweetened almond milk

1 potato, peeled, diced, and cooked

2 cups frozen mixed vegetables, thawed

2 (9-inch) pie crusts (store-bought or homemade)

Preheat your oven or grill (we use a Traeger) to 350°F.

In a large pot, melt the butter over medium heat. Sauté the onion until tender, 5–7 minutes. Add the wild turkey breast and brown, stirring occasionally, for 5–7 minutes. Add the flour, spice rub, pepper, thyme, and rosemary and cook for 2 minutes. Whisk in the chicken stock and milk a little at a time, stirring after each addition. The gravy will start to smooth out after a few minutes of cooking and stirring. Bring to a boil over medium heat, then turn down the heat and simmer for 1–2 minutes. Stir in the vegetables and remove the pot from the heat.

Have ready two 5-inch ceramic ramekins. Roll out the pie crusts to about 12 inches around. Cut out two circles from each pie crust, one a bit larger than the other, both bigger in diameter than the ramekins. Line each ramekin with the larger circle of dough. Spoon the turkey mixture into the lined ramekins until level with the top. Place another circle of dough on top of each filled ramekin as a lid. Pinch the edges all the way around to seal. Cut 3 or 4 slits on top to vent the pies. Bake for 40–45 minutes, until the crust is lightly browned. Let cool for 10 minutes before enjoying.

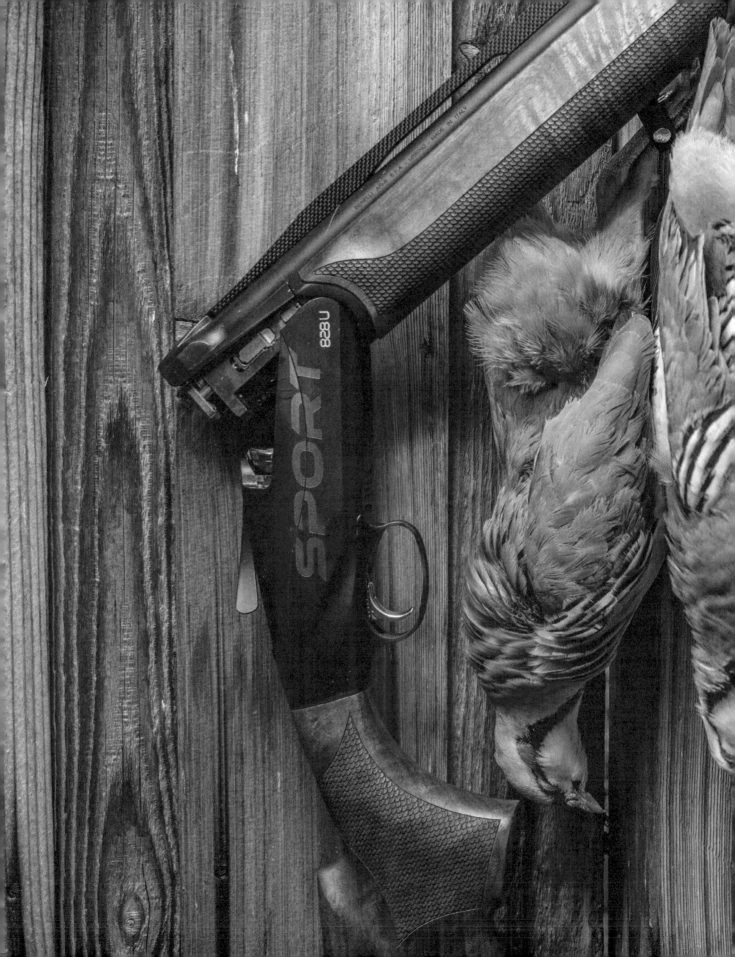

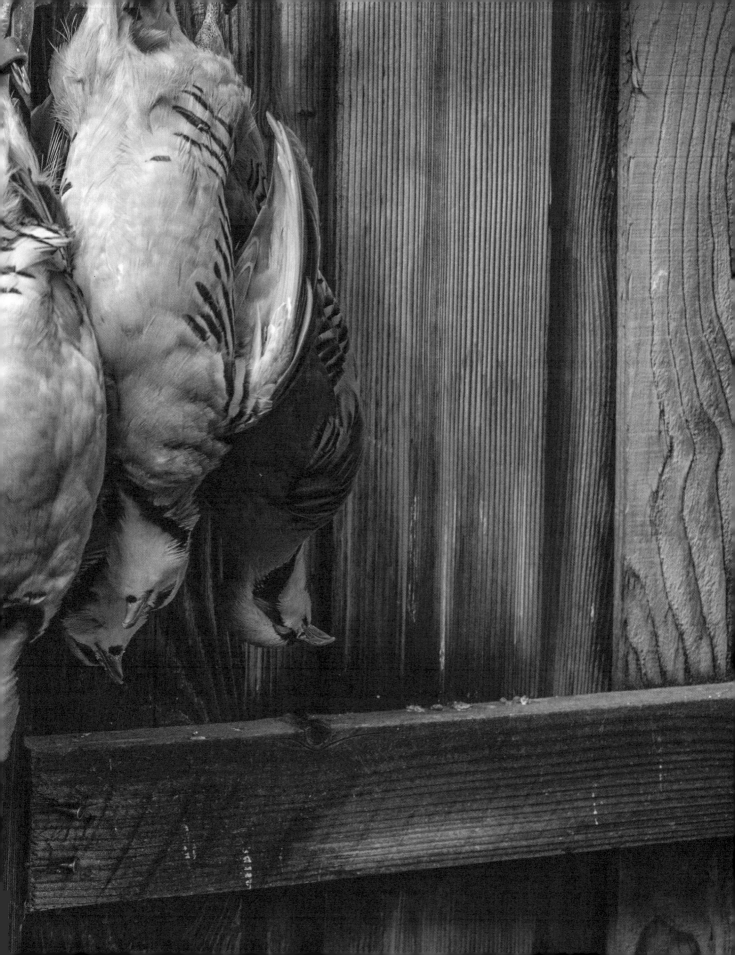

Upland Game Bird in Mushroom Sauce

SERVES 4

Perhaps you've tried other versions of this recipe, but we bet you haven't had upland game bird in mushroom sauce done with love and passion! Put on some country music, pour yourself a glass of white wine, smile, and take your time making it. This flexible recipe works well with smaller birds like chukar, dove, quail, or pheasant. Serve with wild rice, brown rice, or your favorite pasta.

---

2 tablespoons unsalted butter, plus more for greasing

1 tablespoon olive oil

2 upland game birds, boned (about 2 pounds total)

1 yellow onion, sliced

3 garlic cloves, minced

2 cups sliced white mushrooms

Salt and ground black pepper to taste

½ cup dry white wine

1 (10.5-ounce) can condensed cream of mushroom soup

Heat the oven to 350°F. Lightly grease a 2-quart casserole dish with butter.

Melt the 2 tablespoons of butter and the olive oil in a large skillet over medium-high heat. Brown the birds lightly, 2–3 minutes per side. Add the onion, garlic, and mushrooms and sauté lightly until the veggies are soft. Season with salt and pepper.

Using tongs, transfer just the birds to the prepared casserole dish. Add the wine and cream of mushroom soup to the mushroom mixture in the skillet and heat to a slow boil. Pour the mushroom sauce over the birds and cover the casserole dish with a lid or aluminum foil. Bake for 45 minutes, or until the birds are cooked through.

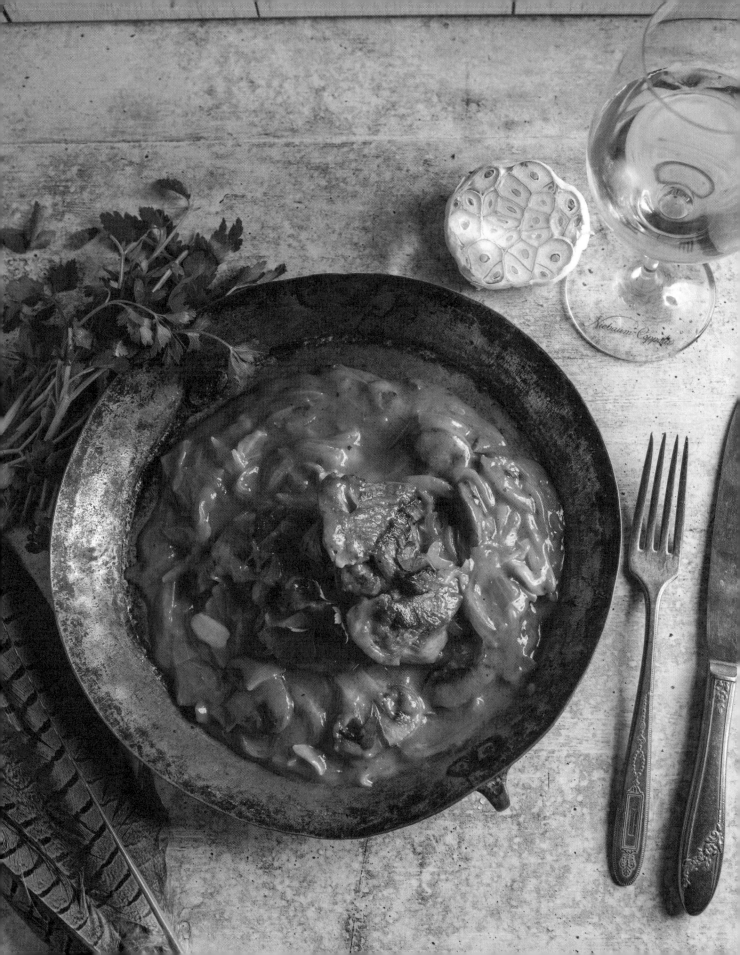

Chukar Joey

SERVES 4–6

This recipe, courtesy of our friend Jim Rhea, was created on a chukar hunting trip in Winnemucca, Nevada. After a long day of hunting, we returned to the "social club" we were staying at. Having been on dusty roads most of the day, we had a few adult beverages to clear our throats while we cleaned our birds. One of our party, a fellow who goes by the name Joey, maybe had a couple too many beverages and went to sleep before dinner was served. We thought it only fitting to name the dish after him.

1 cup all-purpose flour

1 tablespoon salt

1½ teaspoons ground black pepper

1 teaspoon paprika

1 teaspoon garlic powder

6–8 chukar breast fillets (from 3–4 chukars)

3 tablespoons olive oil

3 tablespoons unsalted butter

2 cups chopped bell pepper (any color)

2 shallots, diced

2 cups thinly sliced mushrooms

1 cup 80-proof brandy

4 garlic cloves, minced

1 cup dry white wine

1 cup chicken stock

Juice of ½ lemon

2 tablespoons cornstarch mixed with
    2 tablespoons water (optional)

½ cup chopped fresh chives

1 pound linguine, cooked according to
    package directions

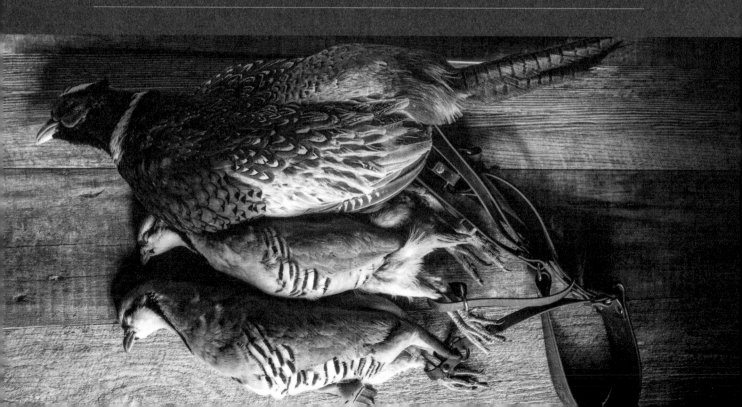

In a 1-gallon resealable plastic bag, combine the flour, salt, black pepper, paprika, and garlic powder. Lightly pound each breast fillet and cut into 2-inch pieces. Add the pieces to the bag with the flour mixture, seal, and shake to evenly coat. Remove from the bag and shake off the excess.

Heat the olive oil and butter in a large cast-iron skillet over medium heat. Brown the chukar pieces for 2–3 minutes per side. Transfer to a plate lined with paper towels.

Add the bell peppers and shallots to the same pan and sauté until the shallots are soft, 1–2 minutes. Stir in the mushrooms. Pour the brandy into the pan with the mushrooms and carefully ignite with a long match to flambé. Once the flames subside, add the garlic and stir for 1 minute, or until fragrant. Add the white wine, chicken stock, and lemon juice and cook until reduced by half. If you'd like your sauce thicker, stir in the optional cornstarch slurry. Once you have a nice thickened sauce, return the chukar to the pan and add the chives. Let simmer for a few minutes to warm the fillets.

Serve over the linguine.

Jim says: "I like to use both red and green bell peppers to give the dish some added color."

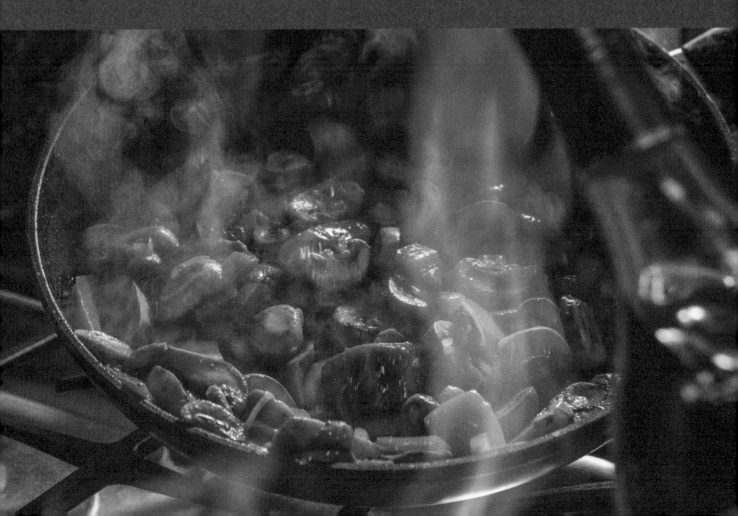

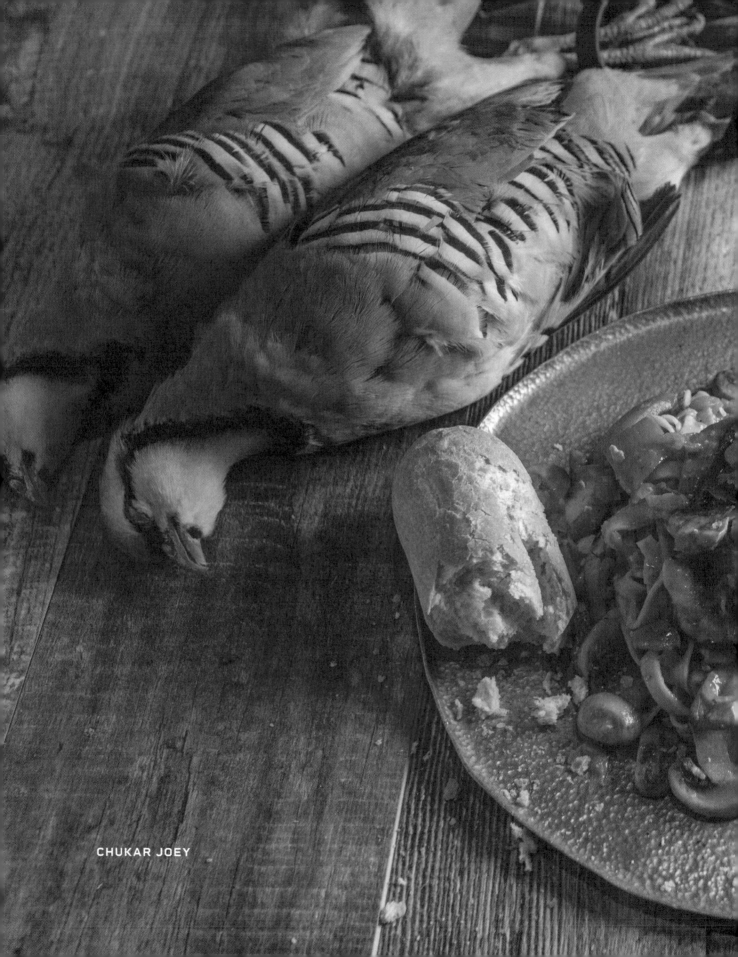

CHUKAR JOEY

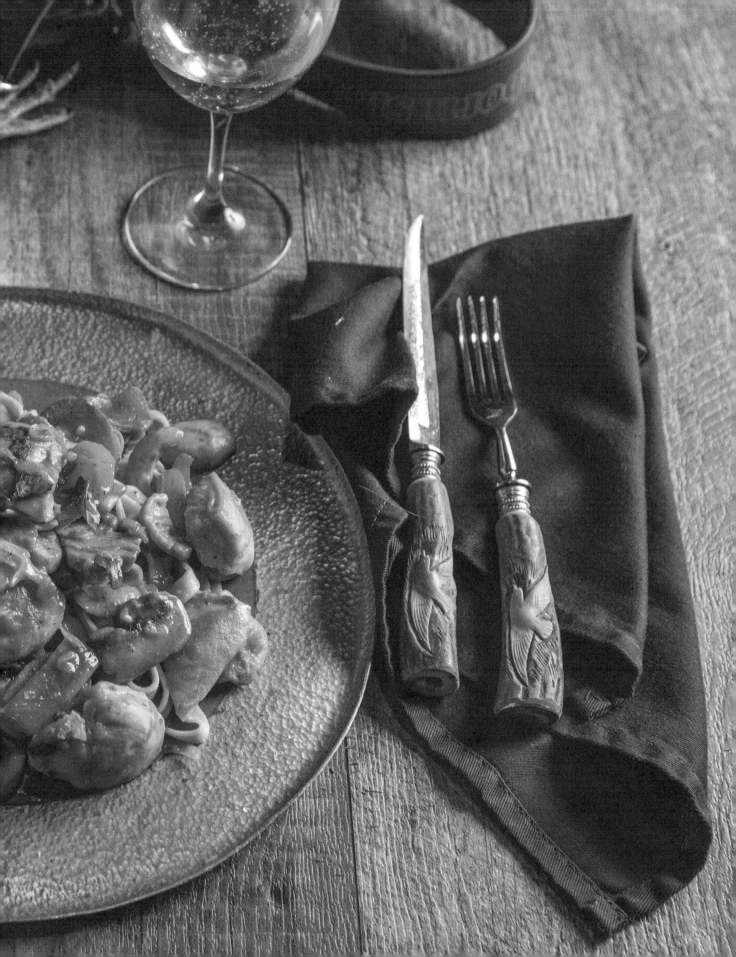

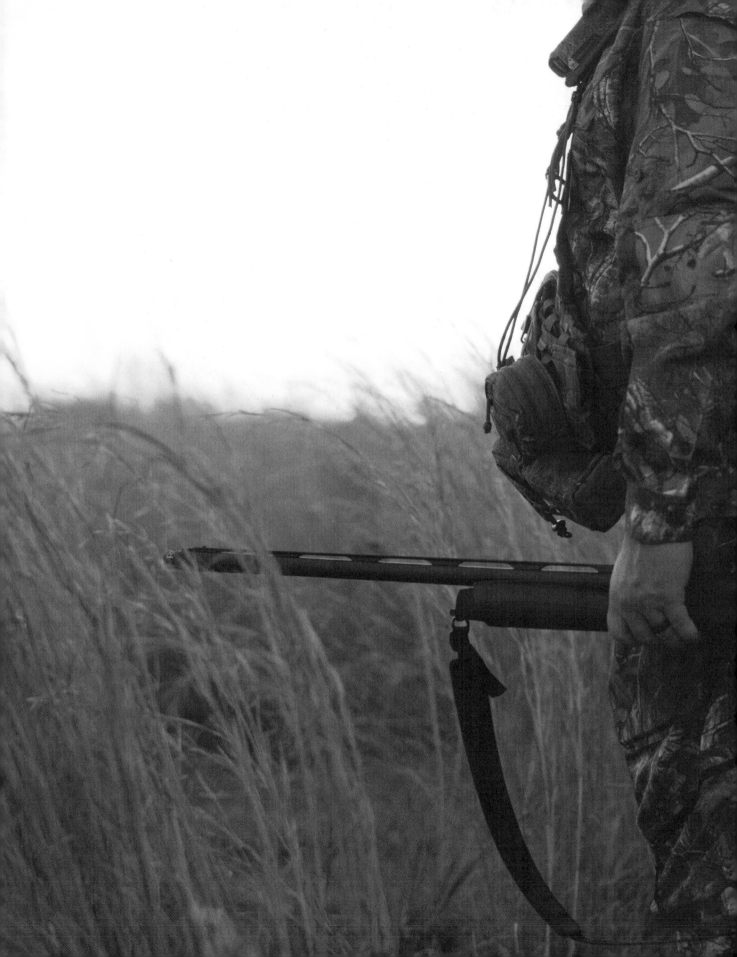

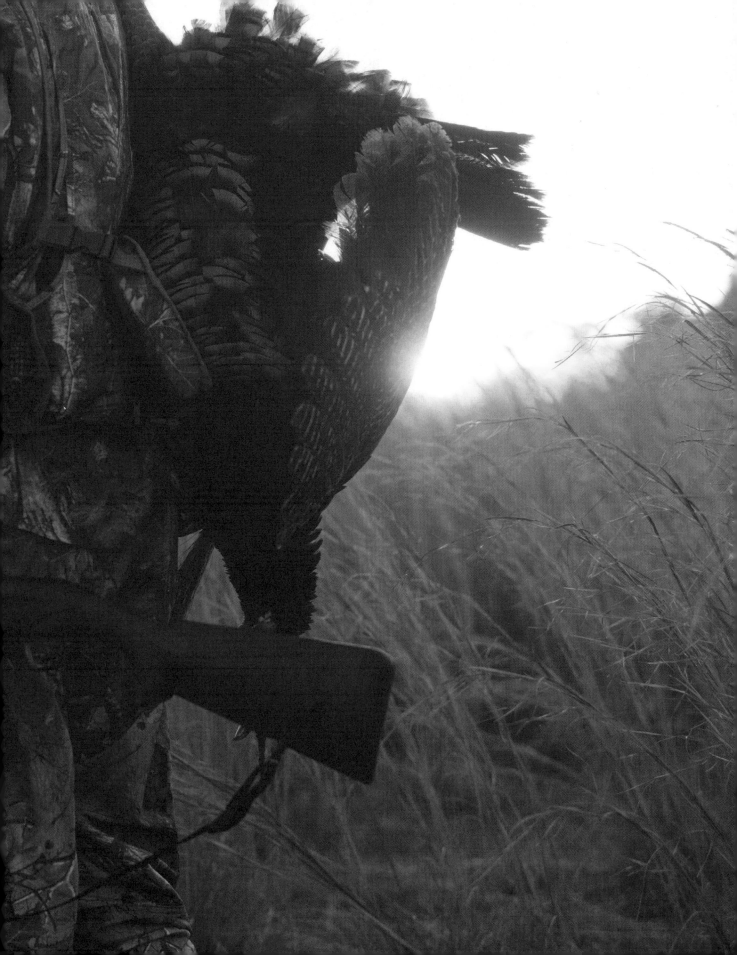

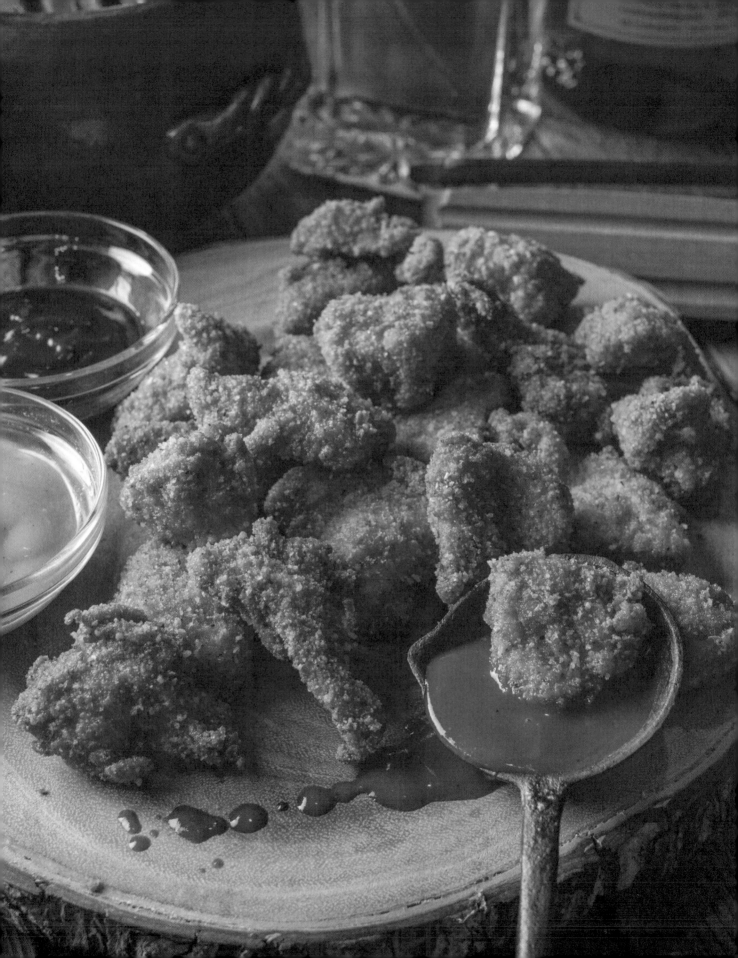

Wild Turkey Nuggets

SERVES 6

Our friend JT Harden has perfected these wild turkey nuggets, a super simple recipe that will please everyone in the family. We highly recommend these tasty nuggets after your next wild turkey harvest! With a mature bird, you'll need half a breast. With a jake or hen, use the whole breast.

½ wild turkey breast (about 2 pounds)

1 (12-ounce) can evaporated milk

3 cups dry bread crumbs

¼ cup Cajun seasoning

1 tablespoon salt

1 tablespoon ground black pepper

Neutral vegetable oil, for frying

Dipping sauce, for serving

Clean and cut all the silverskin and tendons from the turkey breasts. Cut the breasts into bite-size nuggets. Pour the evaporated milk into a large bowl. Add the turkey nuggets and mix until all the nuggets are coated. Cover the bowl with plastic wrap and refrigerate for 4–6 hours.

In a 1-gallon resealable plastic bag, mix the bread crumbs with the Cajun seasoning, salt, and pepper. Remove the nuggets from the refrigerator and drain them. Add the nuggets to the bag, seal, and shake until thoroughly coated in the seasoned bread crumbs.

Pour enough vegetable oil into a large frying pan to cover about half of the nuggets. Heat over medium-high heat until the oil hits 350°F. Add half of the turkey nuggets and cook for 2–3 minutes on each side, until browned and cooked through. Use tongs or a slotted spoon to transfer the cooked nuggets to a plate lined with paper towels. Repeat with the remaining nuggets. Serve with your favorite dipping sauce.

Wild Turkey and Bacon Skewers

SERVES 4

We love wild turkey, honey, bacon, and chili powder, so naturally we had to combine them and add a little smoke flavor from the grill! These skewers are so juicy, and the flavor from the bacon and honey goes great with the kick from the chili powder. With a mature bird, you'll need half a breast. With a jake or hen, use the whole breast.

½ wild turkey breast (about 2 pounds), cut into 1-inch pieces

1 pound thin-sliced bacon

¼ cup honey

1 tablespoon The Provider Fowl Rub or your favorite spice rub

1 tablespoon chili powder

Preheat your grill (we use a Traeger) to 375°F.

Slide the wild turkey pieces onto skewers until each skewer is about full.

Cut each bacon slice into two or three pieces and wrap a piece around each piece of turkey. Lock the ends of the bacon together by piercing with a toothpick.

In a bowl, combine the honey (if it's too thick, microwave it for a few seconds) and spice rub and mix well. Brush the honey mixture all over the turkey and bacon, making sure to get all the sides and crevices. Sprinkle a bit of chili powder over each skewer.

Set the skewers directly on the grill and cook for 15–20 minutes, until the turkey has reached 165°F. Remove and enjoy immediately.

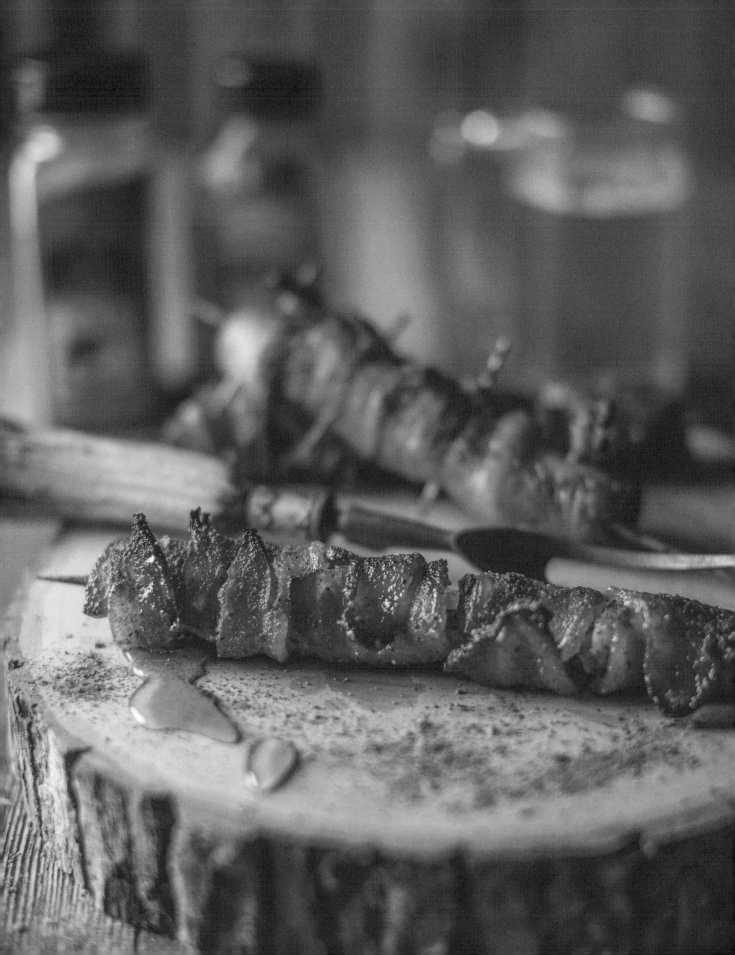

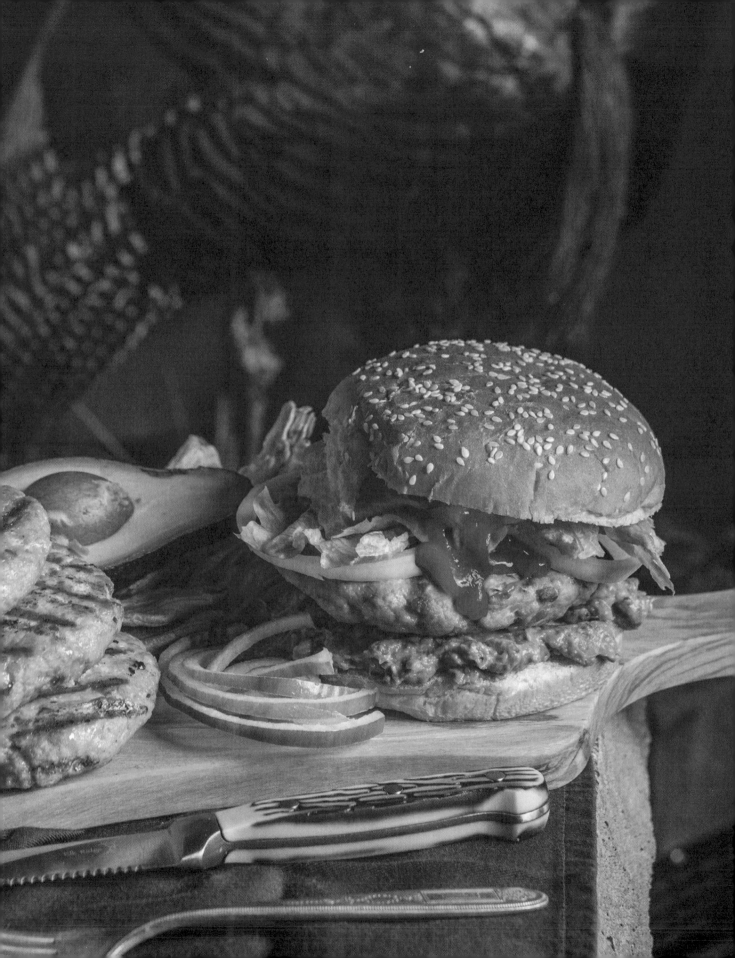

Turkey Guacamole Burgers

SERVES 8

This amazing recipe comes courtesy of Chad Mendes's friend Rihana Cary. It is a creative, healthy, and delicious way to use more of that last wild turkey you harvested. Mixing bacon in with the turkey leaves these burgers juicy and packed full of flavor!

1 pound slab bacon

3 pounds wild turkey

1 tablespoon crushed red pepper

1 tablespoon onion powder

1 teaspoon garlic powder

½ teaspoon paprika

½ teaspoon ground cumin

½ teaspoon salt

½ teaspoon ground black pepper

GUACAMOLE

2 avocados, peeled, pitted, and mashed

1 tablespoon minced garlic

½ cup diced tomatoes

1–2 tablespoons minced red onion

1 tablespoon minced jalapeño

1 tablespoon chopped fresh cilantro

Juice of ½ lime

1 tablespoon crushed red pepper

½ teaspoon ground cumin

Salt to taste

BURGERS

Burger buns

Fresh or pickled sliced jalapeños

Lettuce leaves

Sliced red onions

Ketchup

Preheat your grill (we use a Traeger) to 350°F.

Grind the bacon, then the turkey meat, through your grinder on the ½-inch disk setting. Combine the bacon and turkey and run the mixture through on the ¼-inch disk setting. Add all the seasonings and mix well. Shape into 8 patties.

Cook the patties directly on the grill grate for 10–15 minutes on each side. (Alternatively, you can cook the patties in an oiled cast-iron skillet on the stovetop over medium heat.)

While the burgers are cooking, mix together all the guacamole ingredients in a bowl.

Assemble your burgers on the buns with the guacamole, jalapeños, lettuce, red onion, and ketchup.

Wild Turkey and Rice Soup

SERVES 6–8

This recipe is one of Chad Mendes's favorite things to make the day after Thanksgiving. It's usually a cold day and soup always sounds perfect. He says, "I love this recipe not only because it tastes amazing, but it allows me to utilize the entire turkey. You can get creative with what vegetables you add and it's super easy to make."

---

1 turkey carcass

4 garlic cloves, chopped

2 bay leaves

1 rosemary sprig

2 teaspoons salt

1 teaspoon ground black pepper

2 cups cooked white, wild, or brown rice

1 white onion, chopped

5–8 carrots, chopped

3 cups quartered mushrooms

Lemon wedges, for serving

Put the turkey carcass in a large pot and add enough water to cover. Throw in the garlic, bay leaves, rosemary, salt, and pepper. Bring to a boil over medium heat, then reduce to a simmer and cook for 2–3 hours. Remove the turkey carcass, scraping all the meat into the broth. Fish out any bone pieces that may have come off.

Add the rice, onion, carrots, and mushrooms and cook until the rice is heated through. Remove and discard the bay leaves and rosemary sprig. Ladle the soup into bowls and top with a squeeze of lemon.

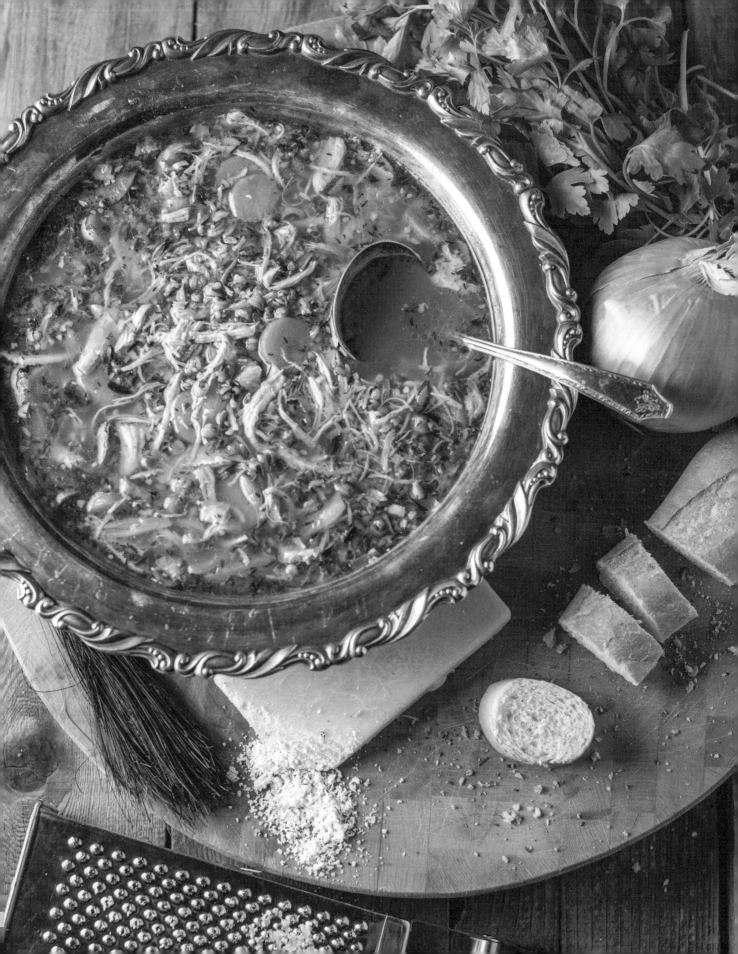

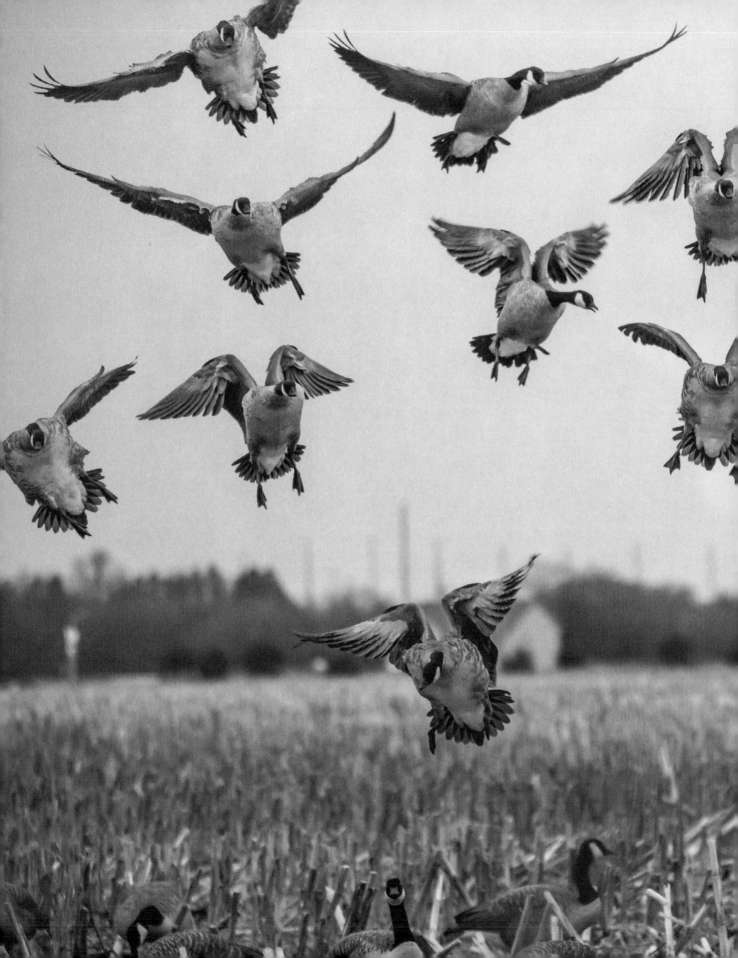

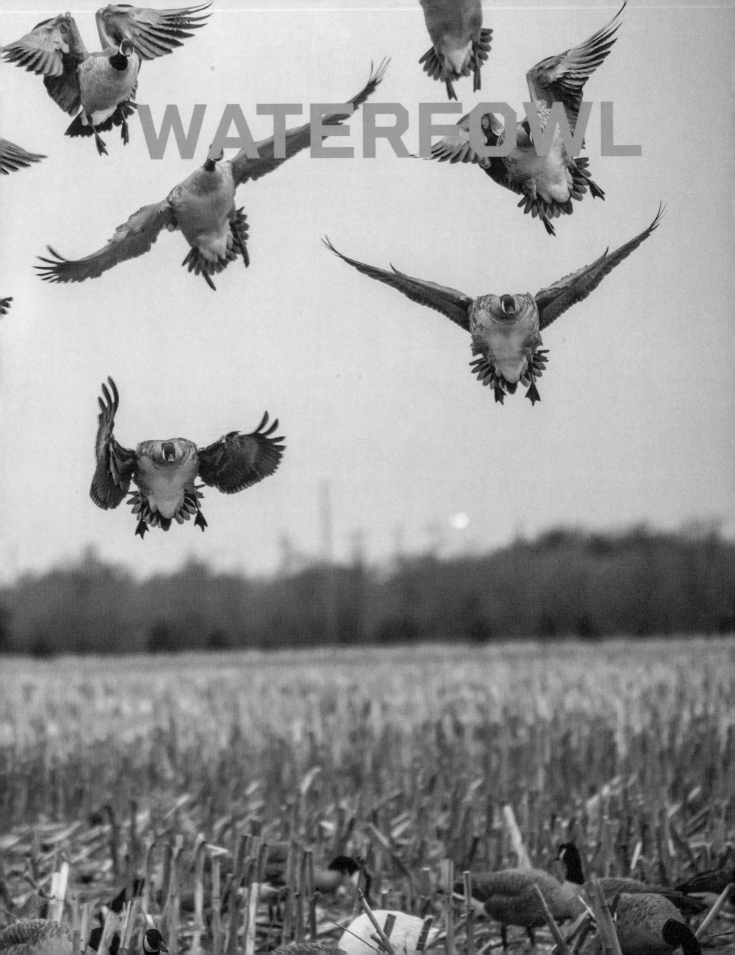

WATERFOWL

There are so many different facets of hunting that draw us to it. It's becoming one with nature; living off the land; studying and understanding wildlife, conservation, and habitat; being at camp with friends and family; and so much more. All of this plays a role in the culture of the waterfowl hunter. Now add the camaraderie in the blind, a duck dog, and communicating with the animals, and you have the complete formula for what draws a man or woman to being a duck hunter!

See, in deer hunting, you are usually by yourself in a tree stand waiting for a deer to walk underneath you. In turkey hunting, you are usually by yourself with your back up against a tree waiting for a tom to approach your decoy. Being by yourself can be cool and even therapeutic. But you aren't by yourself in the duck blind. You are with a group of close friends who are there for the same reasons that you are: to cut up, to tell stories, to make you the butt of their jokes, to cook a meal in the blind, and to keep an eye to the sky for that flock of approaching mallards. Duck hunting is a social event, and that is the draw!

On top of all of this is the study of becoming a more proficient waterfowl hunter. It is gear-intensive, species-specific, and a puzzle that we have to work at relentlessly in order to even begin to put it all together. Waterfowl hunting is a challenge with huge rewards . . . such as a specklebelly goose cooked to medium-rare sitting on a bed of hunter rice and brown gravy. And even when the birds aren't cooperating and it seems like you might go home empty-handed, the duck blind keeps us coming back because we will never get enough of the refrain that takes place within its walls. "Get down, here they come. Get ready . . . get ready . . . take 'em!"

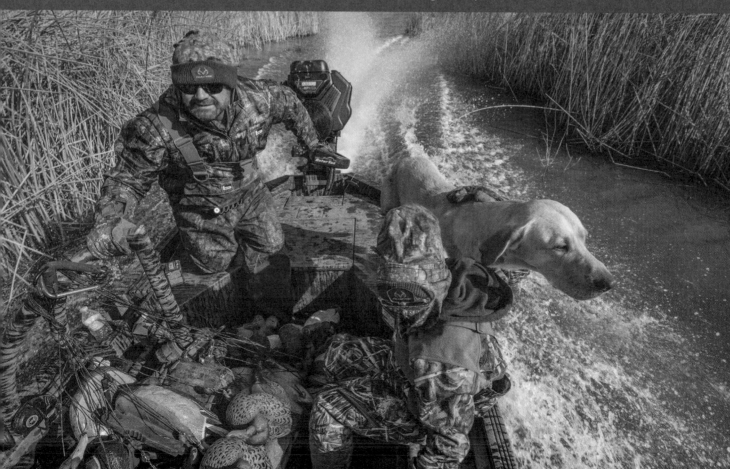

Butchering Wild Fowl

Eating wild fowl is a treat and a delicacy when prepared right. There are so many ways to enjoy it, but first we have to make sure we take care of it from the field to the freezer or table.

We suggest always hanging your ducks or geese from a strap if possible. During the hunt and until you butcher your birds, letting them hang is key.

With ducks and geese, it is OK to remove the breast meat from the body by tearing the skin and fat away to expose the breast fillets. Use the point of a sharp knife to start the cut up against the breast plate. Press the knife to the plate and cut downward as the meat pulls away from the bone. Follow the cut all the way until you are able to separate the bottom of the meat from the skin.

Remember that there is a tenderloin on the duck and goose between the breast fillet and the breast plate. These tenderloins are great for appetizers, so make sure you recognize them and pull them off the breast meat after your cut. We recommend storing your tenders separately from your breast meat.

You can also pluck the feathers away from the skin that covers the breast fillets. This allows you to use the same method above to remove your tenders and breast fillets but leave the skin and fat still on. Then you can crisp up the skin to eat with the meat. When prepared correctly, a bit of duck or goose meat with crispy skin on is possibly the best bite you can have!

You can also pluck the entire bird, which means every feather and pin feather is removed from the bird before freezing. Begin by removing the head and neck, feet, and both wings. Cut an incision in the belly of the bird and remove the entrails. We like to keep the gizzards and the heart for recipes and appetizers. There is also a chance you might have to use a torch to singe some of the small feathers off.

Whether you are plucking the whole bird or just the breast area, it is always a good idea to keep the legs. Legs can be meaty and served as an appetizer or part of the entrée or used in a gumbo roux, gravies, and more.

We suggest vacuum-sealing all of your birds before placing them in the freezer to ensure longer freezer life and better quality.

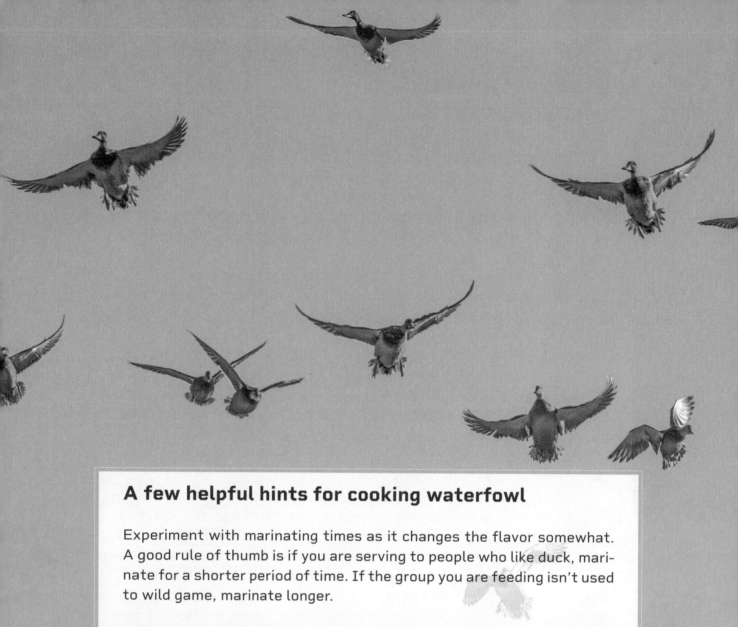

A few helpful hints for cooking waterfowl

Experiment with marinating times as it changes the flavor somewhat. A good rule of thumb is if you are serving to people who like duck, marinate for a shorter period of time. If the group you are feeding isn't used to wild game, marinate longer.

The most common mistake when cooking waterfowl is overcooking it. It then becomes dry and tasteless. Take it off the grill when it is rare or just past rare and it will be perfect.

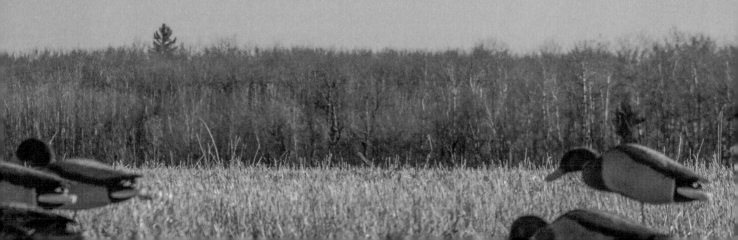

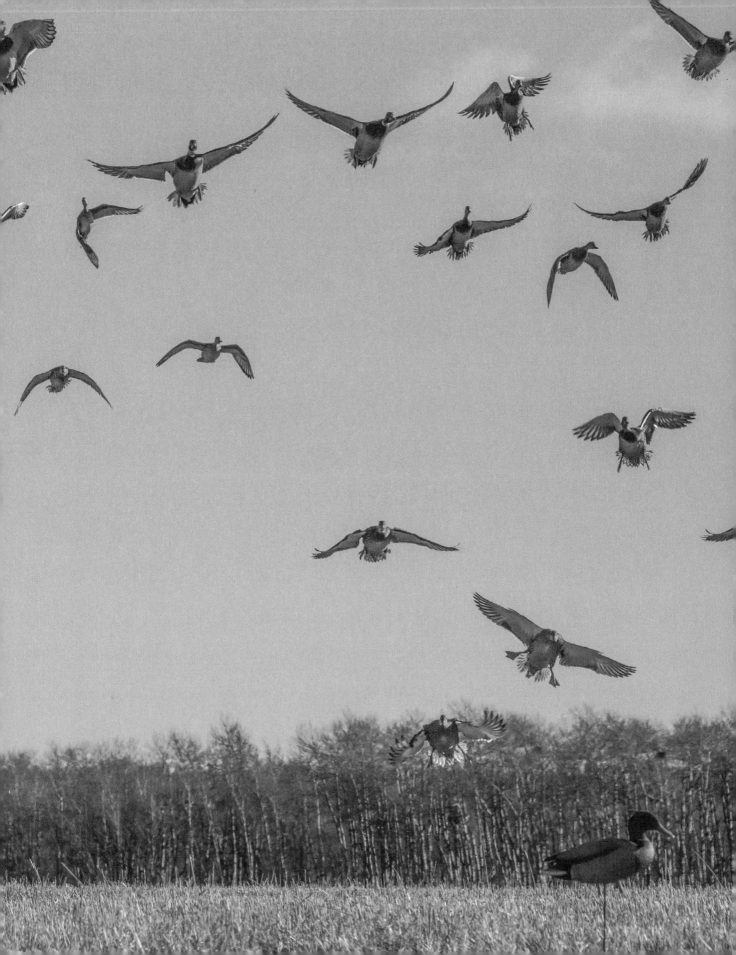

Pulled Goose BBQ Sandwiches

SERVES 4-6

This recipe was designed to use on big Canada geese or old geese in general.

6 boneless, skinless goose breasts

1 gallon apple cider

2–3 tablespoons seasoned salt

2 cups barbecue sauce, or to taste

SANDWICHES

Burger buns

Pickle slices

Sliced green onion

Bring a large pot of water to a boil and boil the goose breasts for 20 minutes, then drain and rinse them well under running water.

Put the breasts in a slow cooker and pour in the apple cider. Cover and cook on low for 7 hours, then switch to high and cook for 1 hour more. Remove the breasts and shred with two forks, much as you would with pulled pork. It is easier to pull the meat when it is hot.

Put the pulled goose meat in a large bowl. Season with the seasoned salt and toss with your favorite barbecue sauce. Pile onto buns and add pickles and green onion to make great sandwiches.

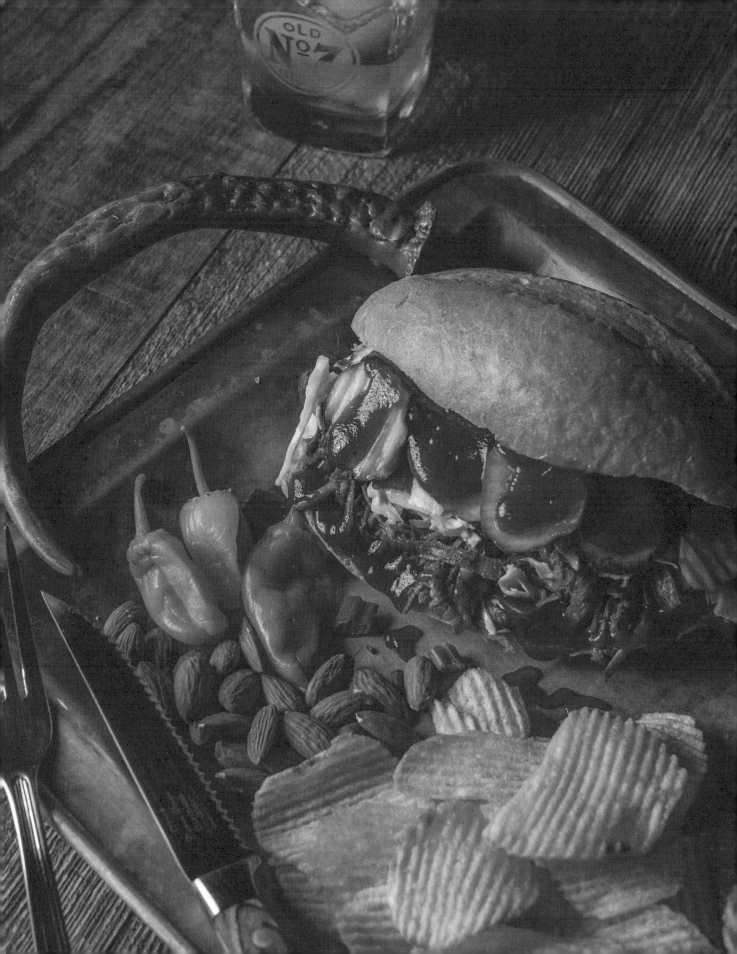

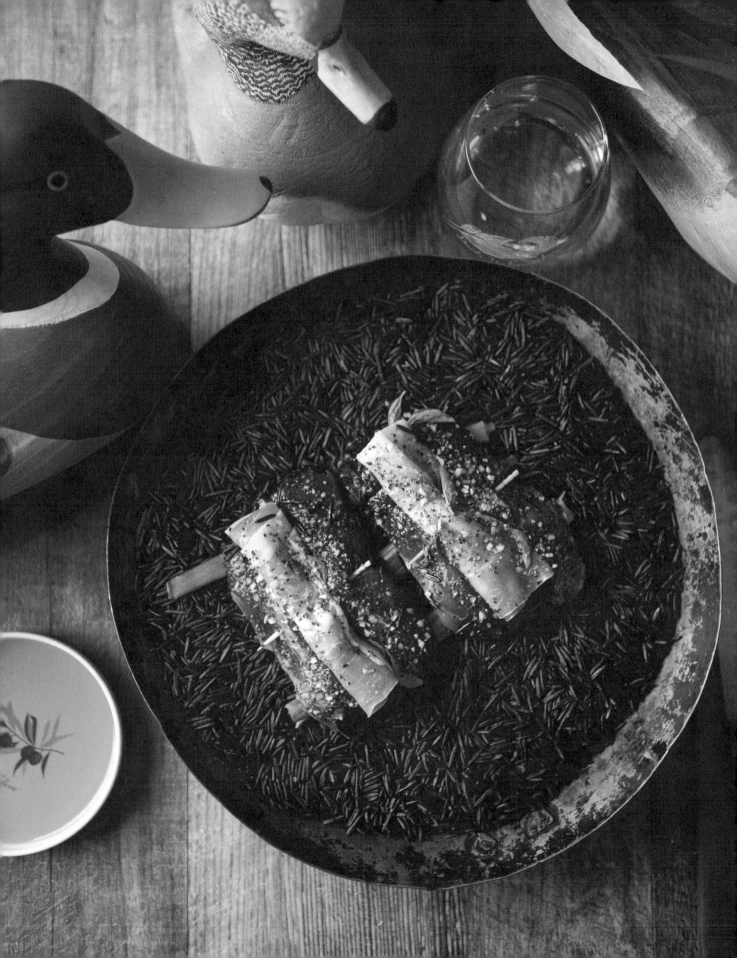

Mamma Del's Duck

SERVES 4

Through his duck-hunting mentor, Dave Stanley, Chad Belding met Paolo Della Bordella, an avid hunter, fisher, and wild game cook. Paolo's mother, Mamma Del, created this dish, which has become a favorite within the hunting community! This recipe works equally well with ducks and smaller geese (specks and snows, especially).

---

4 boneless, skinless duck breasts

4–8 fresh sage leaves

2 ounces fontina cheese, thinly sliced

4 slices prosciutto

1 tablespoon olive oil

2 tablespoons Montreal steak seasoning or your favorite spice rub

---

Preheat your grill (we use a Traeger) to 400°F.

In each breast, cut a deep slit lengthwise on the side that was against the bone to create a pocket. Do not cut all the way through.

Evenly divide the sage leaves, fontina, and prosciutto among the pockets. Use three or four toothpicks to secure the stuffed duck breasts.

Drizzle the oil on the breasts and season with the Montreal steak seasoning.

Grill the stuffed duck breasts for 3–4 minutes on each side. When you take them off the grill, they will continue to cook for a few minutes; you want them rare to medium-rare so that they do not dry out. The USDA recommends cooking duck breast to an internal temperature of 160°F, but we prefer ours at 135°F. To our taste, that is the perfect degree of doneness. Remove the toothpicks before serving.

Pan-Fried Duck

SERVES 4-6

This is a very adaptable recipe. If you don't like teriyaki, use Italian dressing, barbecue sauce, or even buffalo sauce if you like things hot!

---

6 boneless, skinless duck breasts

2 cups teriyaki sauce or your favorite marinade

2 tablespoons The Provider Fowl Rub or your favorite spice rub

1 teaspoon garlic powder

1 teaspoon Dash original salt-free seasoning blend

1 teaspoon ground black pepper

2 tablespoons unsalted butter or olive oil

1½ ounces bourbon

Cut the breasts crosswise into ½-inch-thick strips. If some of the strips are bigger than a comfortable bite, cut them in half.

Put the breast strips in a 1-gallon resealable plastic bag with the teriyaki sauce. Add the spice rub, garlic powder, Dash, and pepper. Seal the bag and shake it up to distribute the marinade and spices. Put the bag in the refrigerator and let the duck marinate for 1–12 hours.

Heat the butter in a large frying pan over medium heat. Empty the contents of the bag into the frying pan and add the shot of bourbon. Cook, stirring occasionally, until the duck pieces are medium-rare, 5–10 minutes. The sauce in the pan should be bubbling lightly, not boiling.

TO SERVE AS AN APPETIZER:
Transfer the duck and sauce to a large bowl. Provide some toothpicks and watch them disappear.

TO SERVE AS A MEAL:
Pour the duck and sauce into a pot of your favorite freshly made rice. Stir thoroughly and serve.

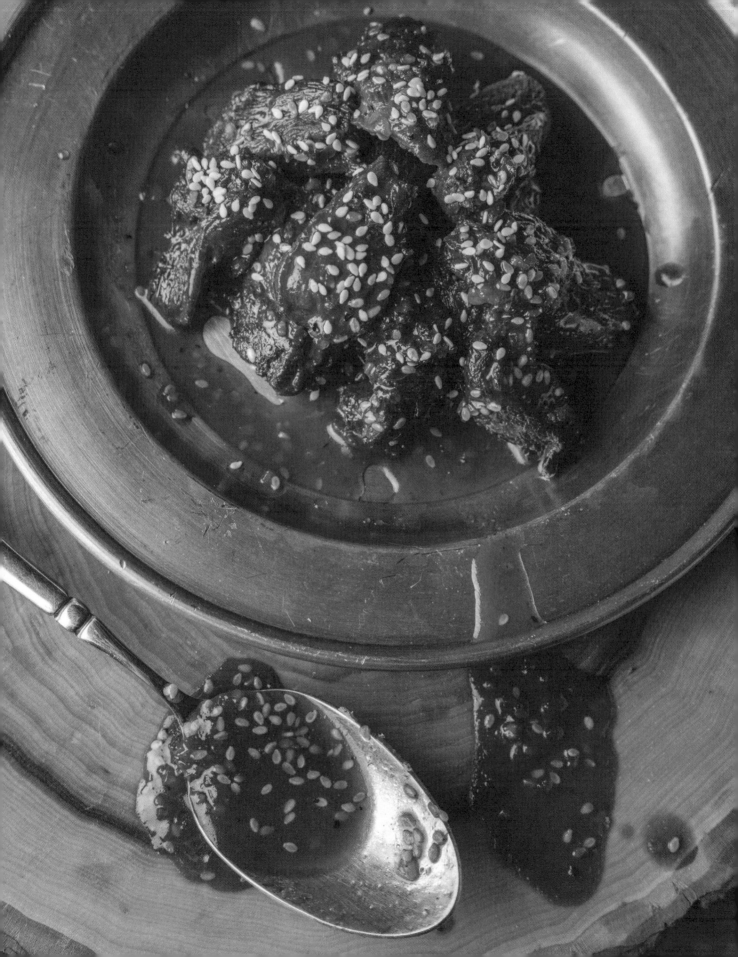

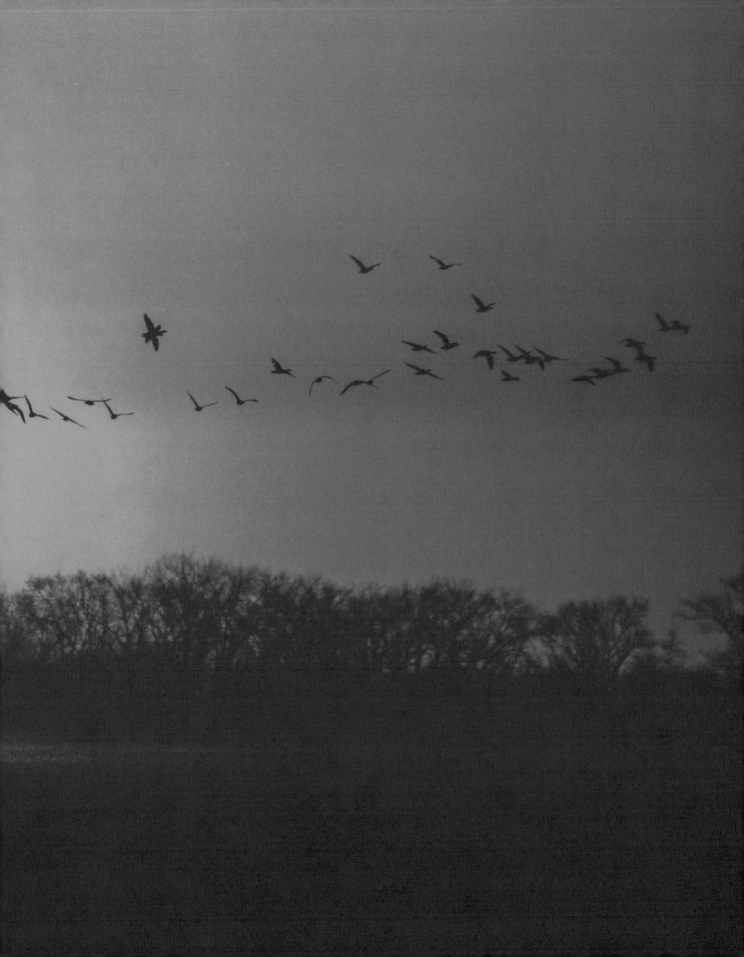

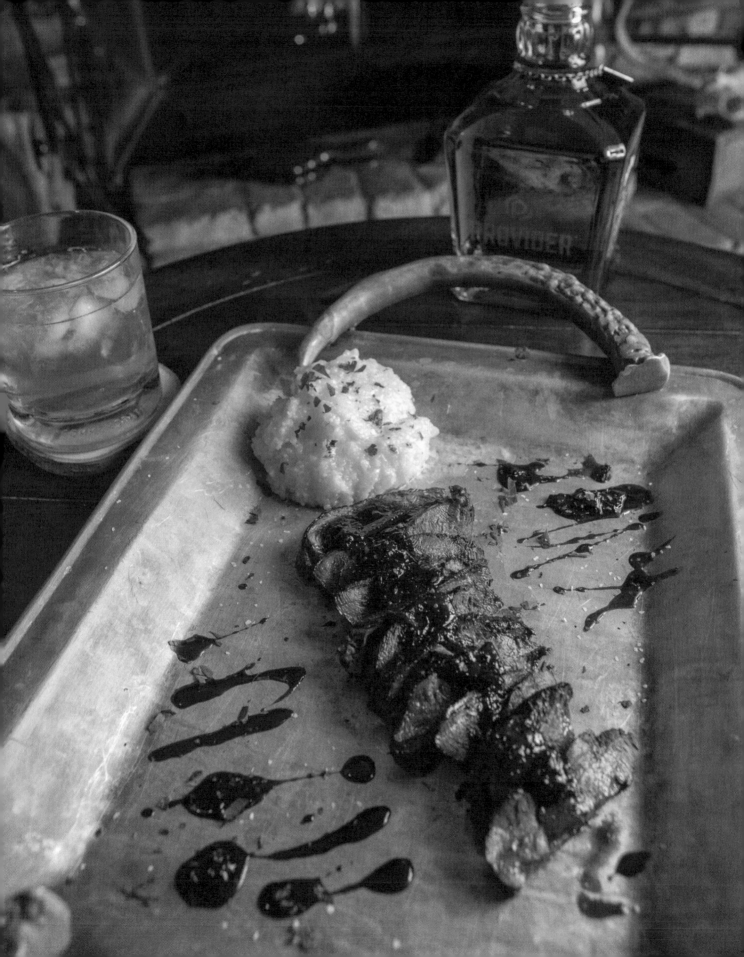

Pan-Seared Specklebelly Goose with Port Wine–Cherry Reduction

SERVES 10

Mike Parker is a master when it comes to putting smiles on his friends' faces through his wild game feasts. Specklebelly goose is one of our favorite wild game meats, and what Mike does with it has us flying high! Pair this dish with your favorite side and a fine wine and believe us, you will be planning your next goose hunt in a hurry! If you can find it, European butter (such as Celles sur Belle brand) is great in this dish because its higher butterfat content imparts extra richness, but any unsalted butter will work. Serve the goose breast and sauce over wild rice, roasted potatoes, or polenta.

6–8 boneless, skin-on goose breast halves

Salt and ground black pepper to taste

⅓ cup balsamic vinegar

⅓ cup brandy

2–3 cups goose stock (recipe follows) or rich
   veal or beef stock

1 cup ruby red port wine

20–25 canned Bing cherries with juice

6–8 tablespoons unsalted butter, cut into
   small pieces

Preheat the oven to 450°F.

Heat a large cast-iron skillet over medium-high heat. Working in batches, place some of the goose breasts, skin-side down, in the skillet. Season with salt and pepper on the meat side. Render the fat from the skin until crisp, about 3–4 minutes. Turn the breasts over and brown the other side for 1–2 minutes. Transfer to a plate, skin-side down.

Add the balsamic vinegar to the fat in the skillet and cook over medium-high heat, whisking frequently, until the fat and vinegar are emulsified and caramelized but not fully sticking to pan. Carefully pour in the brandy, then ignite with a long match to flambé. When the flames subside, reduce the heat to medium. Add the goose stock, port wine, and cherries and cook, stirring occasionally, until the liquid is reduced by roughly two-thirds, 10–12 minutes.

Remove the skillet from the heat. Scatter the butter pieces evenly across the sauce and allow them to slowly melt into the sauce. Whisk until smooth. Season with salt and pepper. Set the skillet

continued

over very low heat to keep warm until ready to serve. (The sauce can be made 1–2 days ahead of serving; if making ahead, refrigerate the seared goose breasts and sauce in separate airtight containers. Allow the breasts to come to room temperature before proceeding with the recipe, and warm the sauce in a small saucepan on the stovetop.)

Arrange the goose breasts, skin-side down, in a large roasting pan (or two, if necessary), leaving at least 1 inch between all breasts and the sides of the pan. Roast the goose breasts for 6–8 minutes for rare/medium-rare.

Plate the goose breasts and spoon the warm sauce generously over them. Serve immediately.

Goose (or Duck) Stock

2 goose (or 4 large duck) carcasses	Salt and ground black pepper to taste
6–8 medium carrots, cut in a few pieces	6–8 rosemary sprigs
6–8 large celery stalks, cut in a few pieces	10–15 thyme sprigs
3–4 medium onions, halved	3–4 bay leaves
2 garlic heads, halved crosswise	1 (750 ml) bottle zinfandel or other dark
⅓–½ cup extra virgin olive oil	red wine

Preheat the oven to 450°F.

Put the goose carcasses in a large roasting pan. Add the carrots, celery, onions, and garlic to the roasting pan. Pour in the olive oil, season with salt and pepper, and toss with a large spoon until everything is coated. Roast, stirring occasionally, until the bones are dark brown, 35–40 minutes.

Transfer the contents of the roasting pan to a large stockpot. Add the rosemary, thyme, bay leaves, and zinfandel. Add enough water to fill the pot to 1–2 inches from the top. Cover and bring to a full boil over high heat. Remove the lid and reduce the heat to a simmer. Let the stock simmer for several hours, until reduced by one-third to one-half.

Remove the pot from the heat. Let the stock cool to room temperature, then strain the stock into containers and refrigerate or freeze for future use. Discard the boiled carcasses and vegetables.

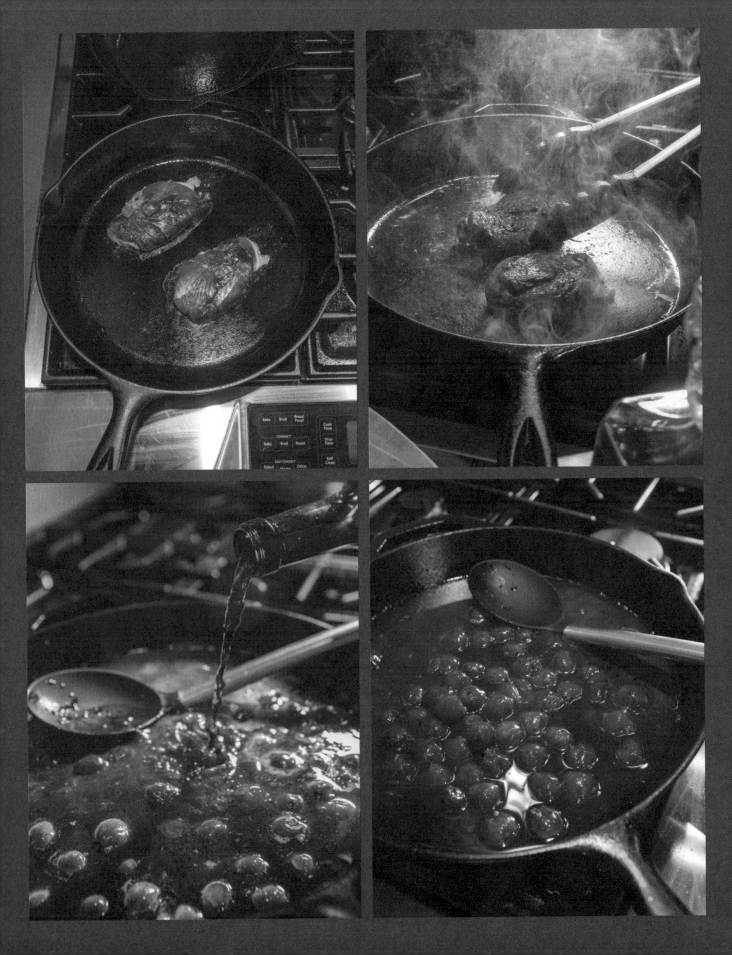

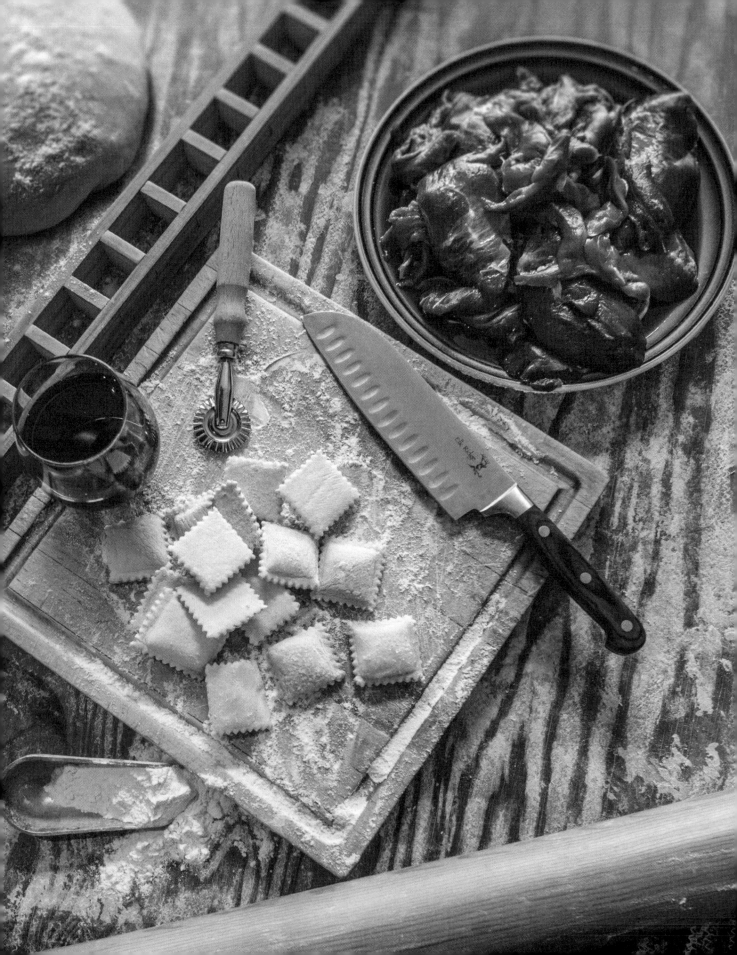

Paul Basso's Ravioli on the Wing

MAKES ABOUT 200 RAVIOLI

Chad Belding's friend Paul loves to bring family and friends together! He has several ways of doing this, but his favorite is with his famous wild duck ravioli. We have been witness not only to the process but also to all of the big smiles around his table. This is a big *recipe—it makes around 200 ravioli. We like to freeze these and pull out only what we need; 6–8 ravioli per person is a great dinner. Making these is an all-day affair, but when you mix that with a little wine and some stories, it goes by way too fast. Salute!*

RAVIOLI FILLING

1 tablespoon olive oil

4 pounds boneless, skinless mallard duck
   breasts, cut into 1-inch pieces

2 teaspoons dried Italian seasoning

Salt and ground black pepper to taste

2 heads iceberg lettuce, cored and quartered

1½ pounds baby spinach

6 large eggs

1½ cups grated parmesan cheese

RAVIOLI PASTA

8 cups all-purpose flour

4 large eggs

2 tablespoons olive oil

2 teaspoons salt

TO SERVE

Paul's Duck Pasta Sauce (recipe follows) or
   your favorite pasta sauce

Grated parmesan cheese

TO MAKE THE RAVIOLI FILLING:

Heat the oil in a large skillet over medium heat. Add the duck, Italian seasoning, and salt and pepper and cook until lightly browned on all sides, about 6 minutes. Remove the pan from the heat.

Bring a large pot of water to a boil. Add the lettuce and spinach and boil until soft, 2–3 minutes. Drain the greens, reserving 6 cups of the cooking water to make the pasta (set it aside to cool). When the greens are cool enough to handle, press out as much water as possible.

In a food grinder, grind the drained cooked greens and cooked duck together into a large bowl. Add the eggs, parmesan cheese, and salt and pepper and mix well.

TO MAKE THE PASTA:

Mound the flour on a clean work surface and make a well in the center. Crack the eggs into the well and add the olive oil and salt. With your hands, break up the eggs and mix everything

continued

together. As the mixture starts to clump together, begin adding the reserved cooled cooking water, ½ cup at a time, and knead until the dough is smooth. Cover the dough with a bowl and let rest for 1 hour.

Divide the dough in half. Using a pasta board and a 3-foot roller, roll the pasta very thin into a circle. Fold the circle in half to make a crease. Unfold and spread half the ravioli filling in a layer ⅛ inch thick over half of the circle. Fold the unfilled half of the circle over the filled side. Press the ravioli using a ravioli press and cut with a ravioli cutter into squares. Repeat with the remaining dough and filling. (At this point you can freeze the ravioli until you are ready to serve; if you're serving right away, count out 6–8 ravioli per person and freeze the rest.)

When you're ready to serve, bring a large pot of water to a boil. Add the desired amount of ravioli to the boiling water and bring the water back to a low boil. Cook, stirring occasionally, until al dente, about 20 minutes.

Warm the sauce gently in a pot. Drain the cooked ravioli and place one layer in a large serving bowl. Add some of the sauce and parmesan cheese and repeat the layers until the bowl is full.

Mangia!

Paul's Duck Pasta Sauce

2 pounds boneless, skinless mallard duck breast, cut into ½-inch pieces

½ cup all-purpose flour

1 tablespoon olive oil

½ large onion, diced

3 garlic cloves, pressed

4 cups water

1 (6-ounce) can tomato paste

1 tablespoon chopped fresh parsley

1 tablespoon fresh rosemary

1–2 teaspoons chili powder

⅛ teaspoon ground allspice

Pinch ground nutmeg

Salt and ground black pepper to taste

Coat the duck pieces with the flour.

In a large Dutch oven, heat the oil over medium heat. Add the duck, onion, and garlic and cook until the duck is browned, about 5 minutes. Add the water, then stir in the tomato paste and all the herbs and spices. Let simmer for at least 1 hour, adding more water as needed to maintain your desired consistency. (For better flavor, make the sauce the day before serving; refrigerate in an airtight container overnight.) This recipe makes enough sauce for 4 servings of ravioli.

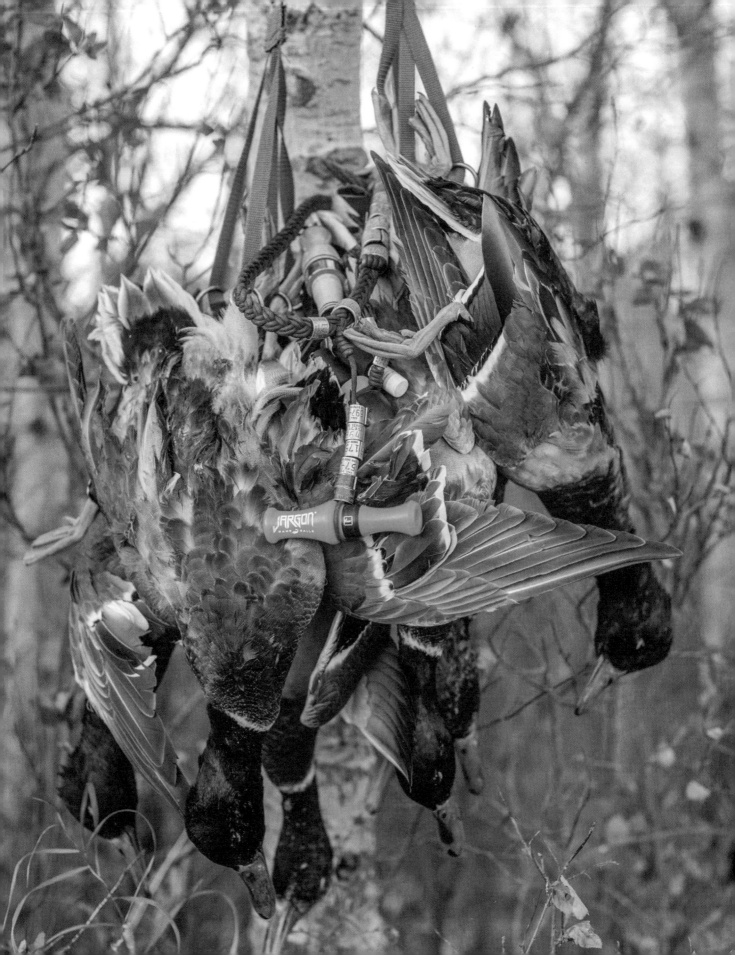

Timber Dreams

Chad Belding

Picture a funnel. Place that funnel over a map of the United States, with the wide part over Montana and North Dakota and the skinny part over the state of Arkansas. Now, fill that funnel with mallard ducks. This is how Arkansas became the Mallard Duck Capital of the World! A vast area funnels down into one location, and many of these mallards end up there. Welcome to the Grand Prairie!

If you ask any duck hunter, they will tell you that it is their dream to hunt in Arkansas. It's a quiet area because at one time it was all timber. Then rice farming became profitable. Thousands of acres of trees were cleared, and rice fields were planted. With an ample food source and havens of tall pin oak trees that still existed in patches, a kind of Duck Disneyland was born.

The mallards figured out the perfect way to capitalize on their new menu. They would eat in the rice fields all night, then return to the security blanket of flooded timber trees to spend their days. These trees kept birds of prey away, and acorns would drop and become the ducks' dessert after a belly full of rice. So then, duck hunters figured, heck, let's go into the timber.

Flooded timber duck hunting can be as powerful and memorable an experience as anything a hunter could ever witness. Five ducks can turn into a hundred ducks in a matter of seconds, and they descend from high altitudes to the timber patches. Hunters use the trees as a hide, standing up against them, always on the shaded side. A timber hunter always wants the sky to be sunny and the temperatures to be chilly. With the sun, shadows and brightness make it almost impossible for ducks not to parachute into the timber. Take those elements and add duck calls to the mix, and you got yourself a hunt!

The best duck callers in the world hail from Arkansas, and here's why: You have to be able to operate a duck call and sound just like a mallard duck, because with the trees providing a canopy over the water holes, it's difficult for ducks to see other ducks (or hunters' decoys). They follow the sounds to where other ducks are—or the sounds of duck calls to where the duck hunters are! From a young age, duck hunters in Arkansas learn that they will need to rely on authentic sounds in order to be successful in the flooded woods. So this taught us that if we are going to travel to Arkansas, we better have our duck calling game polished.

Arkansas has provided us with so many stories and memories of watching mallard ducks pitch into the trees while we patiently awaited their arrival. We would kick the water to create movement and sounds that the ducks find comfort in, then play peekaboo from one side of the tree to the other depending on where the flocks were approaching from. And when it all came together, it was pure mallard magic!

From the boat rides to the sounds of nature to the wet dogs to the blue skies to the tall pin oak trees to the abundance of wild mallard ducks to historic duck camps to the nicest folks on Earth, Arkansas is the land of the ducks and a welcoming home to any duck hunter.

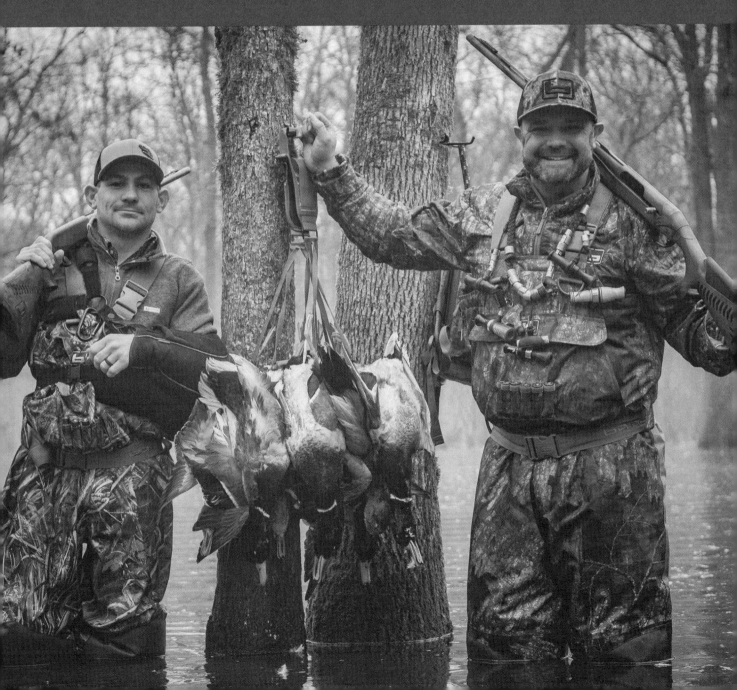

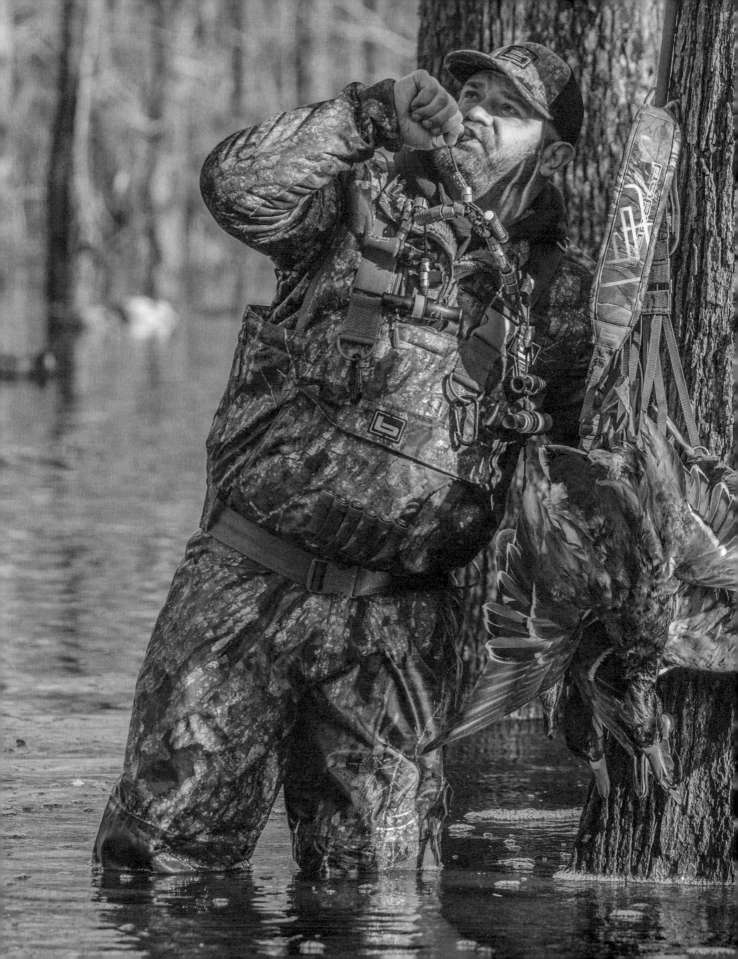

Duck Calling Tips

When choosing a duck call, pick one based on the terrain you will be hunting and on your level of expertise with a call. A loud, high-pitched call will carry long distances, so that's good for open-water hunting. In flooded timber hunts like in Arkansas, pick a softer call. Double-reed calls are easier to control than single-reed calls.

Different hand positions on the end of the call, such as opening and closing your hands, will help you achieve different sounds.

In order to create a perfect seal, position your lips on the mouthpiece exactly as if you would be drinking from a soda bottle. Your tongue will stay positioned at the bottom of your mouth with your jaw moving up and down, controlling the flow of air. Push hot clean air through the call straight from your diaphragm just as you would blow air to fog a window on a cold winter day.

To produce a quack, say either *Hut* or *Oot*, but don't actually enunciate it—what's important is bringing good hot air up from your diaphragm, not pronouncing or adding voice into the call. Think like a quarterback calling "Hut hut!"

Put together a series of single quacks for different cadence:

A greeting is performed by blowing five or six single quacks together in a rhythm. *Hut-Hut-Hut-Hut-Hut-Hut* or *Oot-Oot-Oot-Oot-Oot!*

For a feed call, say (but don't enunciate) *Ka-Ka-Ka-Ka* or *Ticka-Ticka-Ticka-Ticka* into the call.

Always watch the response you receive from the birds for each call you make and adjust accordingly. Once you get a good reaction, let the ducks decide their next move. Don't call too much if they're already on their way in.

Duck Egg Rolls

MAKES 12 EGG ROLLS

Chad Belding's passion for duck hunting started later in life. Growing up in Nevada offered more chances at big game or upland birds. It wasn't until his late twenties that he became addicted to waterfowl hunting. "It all started when I saw a flock of gadwall ducks respond to what I would later learn to be a 'come back' call," he says. "My friend Jim called at them with his duck call, and as soon as they heard it, they spun on a dime and made their way into our decoy spread and, therefore, into our bellies! There was just something about the camaraderie, and the camp life, and the strategy, and the dogs, and the habitat, and the communication between man and bird. Waterfowling would become the basis of everything I would grow into as a man, a businessman, and a Provider!" This tasty recipe comes to us courtesy of Kristy Crabtree from NevadaFoodies.com.

DUCK MARINADE

1 tablespoon soy sauce

1 tablespoon hoisin sauce

1 teaspoon rice wine vinegar

2 teaspoons grated fresh ginger

2 garlic cloves, minced

4 boneless, skinless duck breasts

EGG ROLLS

1 tablespoon olive oil

½ cup chicken stock or water

2 cups finely shredded napa cabbage

1 small red bell pepper, finely chopped

1 carrot, finely chopped

6 green onions, finely chopped

1 cup bean sprouts, chopped

1 (8-ounce) can bamboo shoots, drained and chopped

1 (8-ounce) can sliced water chestnuts, drained and chopped

1 (1-pound) package egg roll wrappers

2 cups canola oil

Sweet chili sauce, sweet and sour sauce, and hot mustard, for serving

---

Combine all the marinade ingredients in a medium bowl and mix well. Add the duck breasts and toss to coat. Cover and refrigerate for at least 1 hour or overnight.

Remove the duck breasts from the marinade and cut into small pieces. Heat the olive oil in a large skillet over medium heat. When the oil is hot, add the duck and cook just until browned and cooked through, 3–4 minutes. Transfer the duck to a bowl and set aside. Add the chicken stock to the skillet along with all the vegetables. Cover the pan and let the vegetables steam for about 5 minutes, until softened. Remove the pan from the heat and drain off the liquid. Add the cooked duck meat to the veggies.

On a cutting board, place one egg roll wrapper with a corner pointed toward you. Place a few tablespoons of the duck and vegetable mixture in the center of the egg roll and fold the bottom corner up over the mixture. Fold the left and right corners toward the center to seal the sides and continue to roll. With your finger, brush a bit of the water on the final corner to help seal the egg roll. Repeat with the remaining wrappers and filling.

Pour the canola oil into a deep pot and heat over medium-high heat to 350°F. Carefully fry 3–4 egg rolls at a time, turning, until golden brown, 3–4 minutes. Remove the egg rolls from the oil and drain on a plate lined with paper towels. Serve warm with sweet chili sauce, sweet and sour sauce, and hot mustard, for dipping.

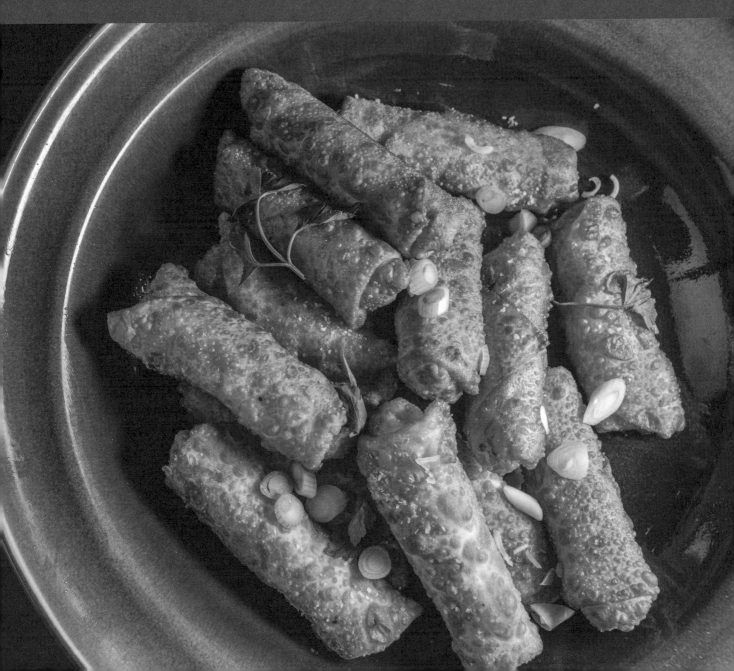

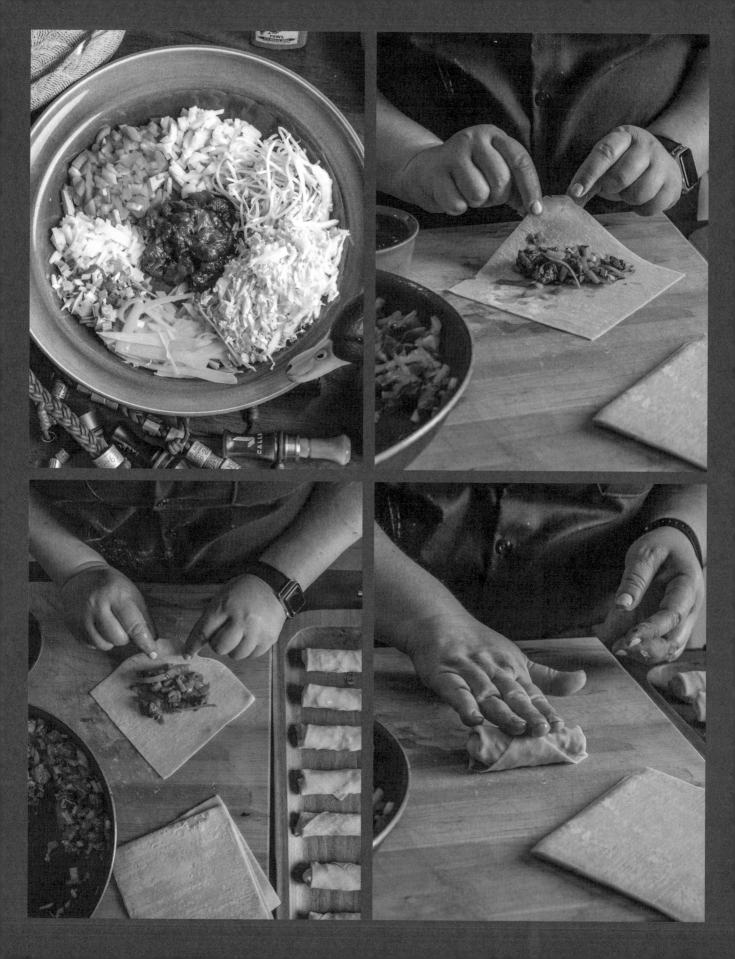

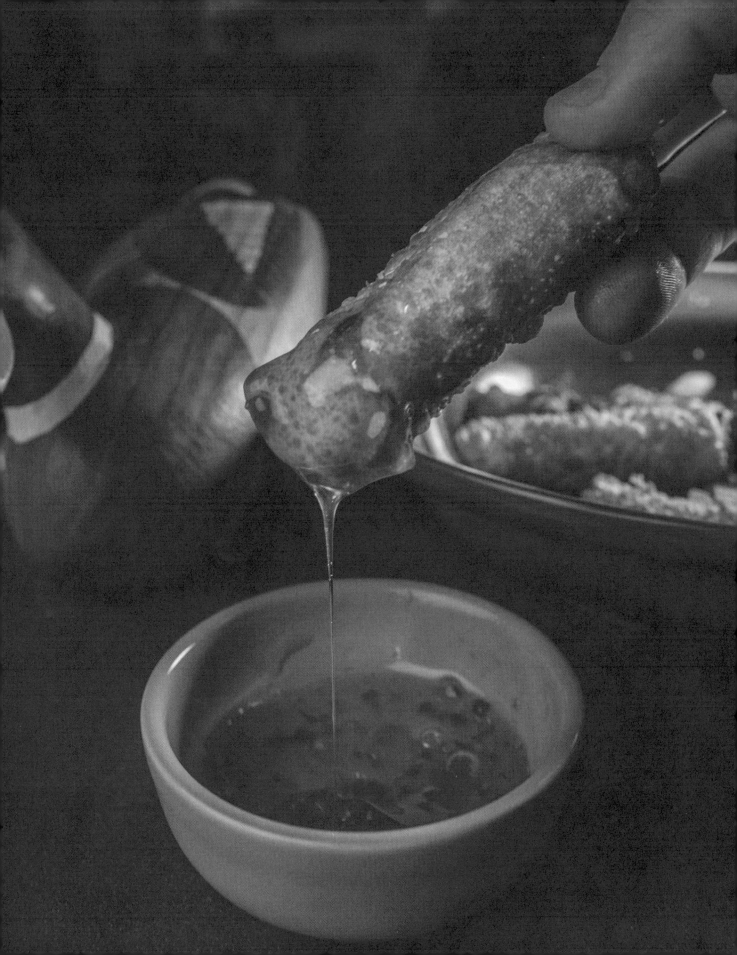

The Snake Mallards

Chad Belding

If you want good potatoes, they say you should go to Idaho. If you want snow skiing, you can find that in Idaho too. If you want a legitimate deer or elk hunt, well, that can be found in Idaho. And then one day, someone told me, if you want mallard ducks, you should head to Idaho for those as well.

I didn't believe it. I even argued a little. Idaho didn't have ducks. No way. But boy, was I wrong! Idaho is like a western corn belt. And where there's corn, you will more than likely find mallards.

My brothers, our friend, and I made the trek to Idaho to chase mallard ducks for the first time in 2008. We had aspirations of hunting the historic Snake River. Long boat rides. Winding waters. Steep canyon walls. It was a fishing river. A boating river. A river to provide water to farmers throughout this area. Everything about it was beautiful, but nothing about it screamed out mallard ducks. And then we came around a turn that headed us to the west and all of a sudden there was an explosion of wings. There were thousands of them, all elevating themselves at the same time to move out of our way. No! They weren't in our way!

They were glorious! Heck, we were in their way. Either way, we found them. And this is where we would return the next morning to set our spread and wait for them to return. It was about to go down.

That night I tossed and turned thinking about how our hunt would play out. Finally the alarm clock, which I didn't need, went off. I was dressed in a flash and my truck was out of the driveway to meet the rest of the guys at the corner store. As we loaded up on unhealthy snacks and coffee, we couldn't help but keep looking at each other and grinning. We knew we had found our gold mine, and now it was time to put our skills to the test. It would be another long boat ride—only this time it was cold, and it was in the dark. We had marked our coordinates, so as long as our GPS was charged up, we were good to go. The boat was loaded down with four men, a more than excited black lab named Axl, three bags of decoys, gun cases, snacks, thermoses, and some five-gallon buckets that would soon become our blind chairs. We were off!

After what seemed like a two-hour boat ride (actually more like 25 minutes—it's always longer when you're excited to get there), we found our spot. Nobody else was there—so far, so good! We each knew what our job was to ensure we were ready when the mallards decided to make their epic return to our marked location. I was in charge of the decoy spread. Clay would be our blind builder. Clint would key in on the dog hide. And Alex would get all of our gear unwrapped from the cases and ready to go to work. We told ourselves that 9:00 a.m. would be the beginning of our mallard dreams coming true.

Anticipation was at an all-time high as the small hand on our watches crept toward that number nine. And just as we envisioned, the mallards came over the big canyon plateau as they left the dry corn fields and pitched down from hundreds of feet up. It was as if they each had their own little parachute on. We called to them and pulled the jerk string. We reached for our Benelli guns. After the smoke settled, all I had to do was say "Axl," and he took off at a dead run until he hit the deeper water. He swam with and against the current to retrieve each mallard duck and return them to us. As we placed them on our straps, we were high-fiving like we just won the state championship. We had done it! We came to the Snake. We scouted the Snake. We found them on the Snake. We returned to where we knew they wanted to be on the Snake. And now we were leaving the Snake with a boat full of green-headed mallards and our heads full of memories.

Now we never let duck season pass without a trip to the Snake River. Every visit is different! Every flock of mallards is just as special as that first one in 2008. One thing that will never change is how all four of us still laugh when people try to tell us that there aren't mallard ducks in Idaho!

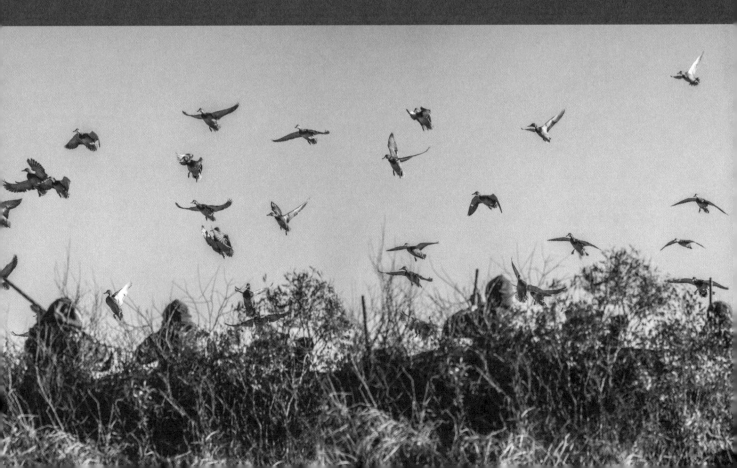

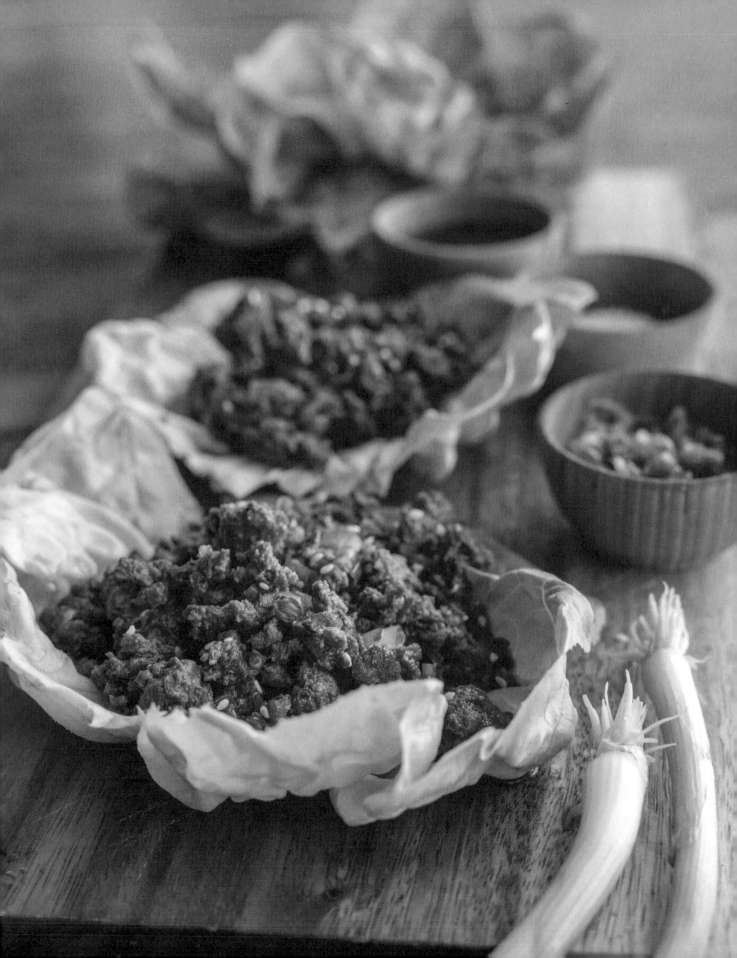

Goose Lettuce Wraps

SERVES 4-6

Running out of ideas for cooking goose? This recipe works great as an appetizer or entrée and will have your guests talking about it for days!

---

1 tablespoon olive oil

1½ pounds ground goose meat (see note)

½ cup finely chopped sweet onion

⅓ cup brown sugar

¼ cup hoisin sauce

2 tablespoons toasted sesame oil

1 tablespoon rice wine vinegar

1 tablespoon soy sauce

2 garlic cloves, minced

1 head butter lettuce

⅓ cup chopped green onion

1 tablespoon sesame seeds

Heat the olive oil in a large skillet over medium-high heat. Brown the goose for 3–5 minutes. Transfer the cooked meat to a bowl. Add the sweet onion to the same skillet and sauté until tender, 5–10 minutes. Stir in the brown sugar, hoisin sauce, sesame oil, rice wine vinegar, soy sauce, garlic, and goose. Stir and cook for 2–5 minutes, until the sauce thickens slightly.

Arrange lettuce leaves around the outer edge of a large serving dish and pile the meat in the middle. Top the meat with the green onion and sesame seeds. Allow everyone to assemble their own wraps and enjoy!

Note: Cubed or finely chopped goose breast can be used instead of ground goose meat.

Goose Potstickers

MAKES 40–50 POTSTICKERS

There are so many ways to enjoy wild goose and we enjoy them all. At the end of the season, when we have built up our inventory of wild meats, we love to get creative with our recipes. This is a takeout-inspired recipe from our good friend Kristy Crabtree of NevadaFoodies.com.

DIPPING SAUCE

1 cup soy sauce

1 tablespoon red wine vinegar

1 tablespoon sugar

1 teaspoon chili sauce

1 teaspoon minced fresh ginger

1 garlic clove, minced

POTSTICKERS

2 boneless, skinless goose breasts, cut into
   1-inch chunks

1 (8-ounce) can water chestnuts, drained

1 (8-ounce) can bamboo shoots, drained

4 green onions, roughly chopped

1 large shallot, roughly chopped

2–3 garlic cloves, peeled

1 tablespoon chopped fresh ginger

1 tablespoon soy sauce

1 tablespoon hoisin sauce

1 teaspoon rice wine vinegar

1 (12-ounce) package potsticker or dumpling
   wrappers

2 tablespoons vegetable oil, divided

1 cup chicken stock, divided

Preheat the oven to 250°F.

In a small bowl, combine all the dipping sauce ingredients and whisk well to combine.

In a food processor, combine the goose breasts, water chestnuts, bamboo shoots, green onions, shallot, garlic, ginger, soy sauce, hoisin sauce, and rice wine vinegar. Pulse until a fine meat stuffing is formed.

To form the dumplings, remove 1 potsticker wrapper from the package and cover the others with a damp cloth. Brush the edges of the wrapper lightly with water. Place a rounded teaspoon of the meat mixture in the center of the wrapper. Fold over, seal the edges, and shape as desired. Set on a rimmed baking sheet and cover with a damp cloth. Repeat until all of the filling is gone.

continued

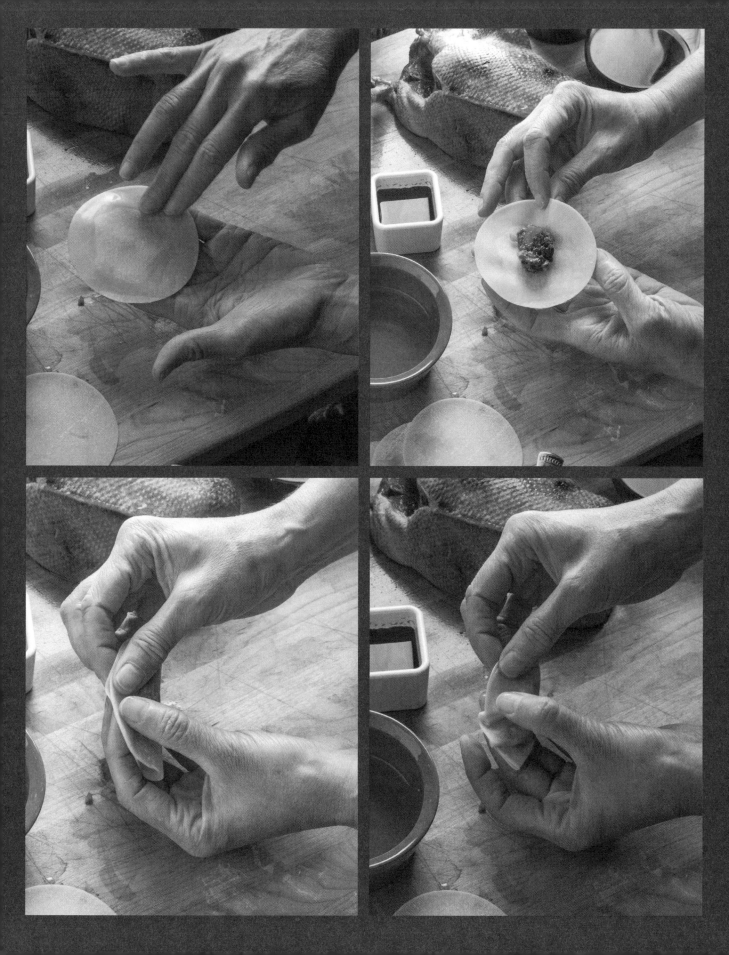

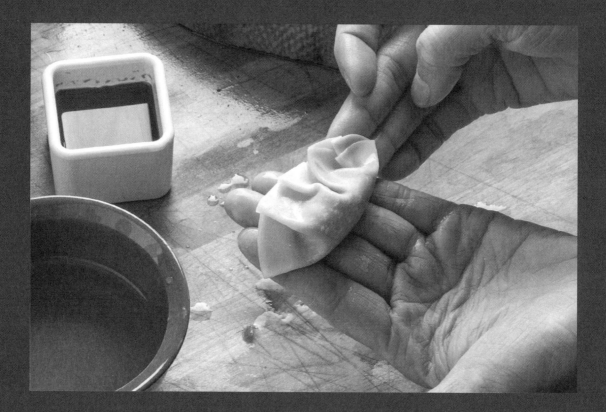

Heat a 12-inch sauté pan over medium heat. Once hot, add about ½ tablespoon of the vegetable oil. Add about 10 potstickers and cook for 2 minutes undisturbed. Gently pour in ¼ cup of the chicken stock, turn the heat down to low, cover, and steam for 2 minutes. Transfer the potstickers to a heatproof platter and place in the warm oven. Clean the pan in between batches and repeat until all the potstickers are cooked. Serve immediately.

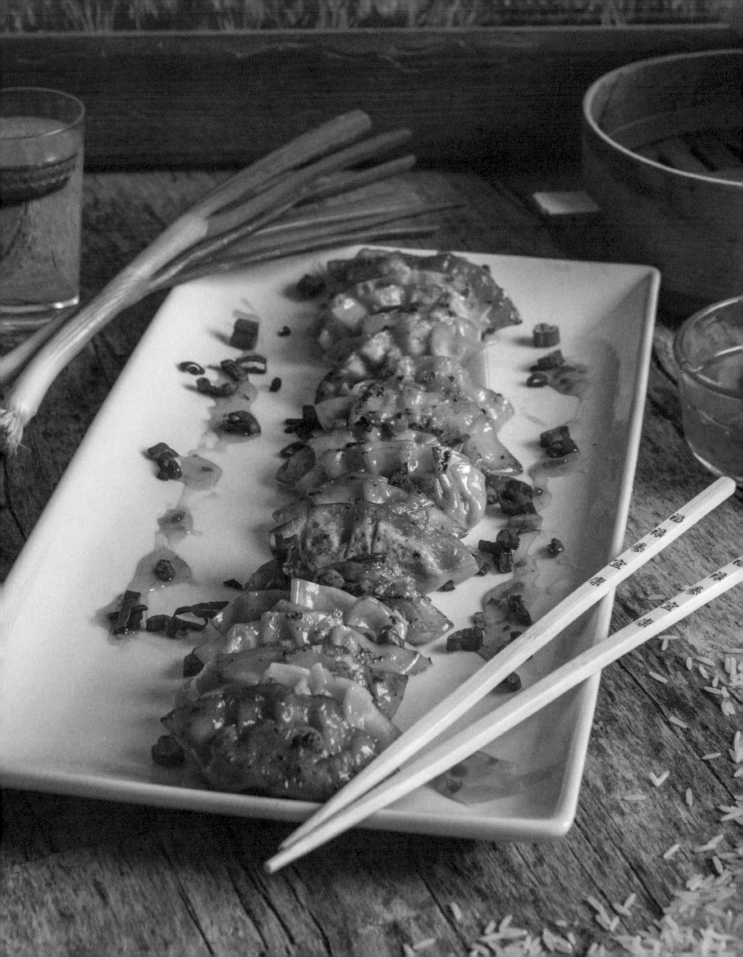

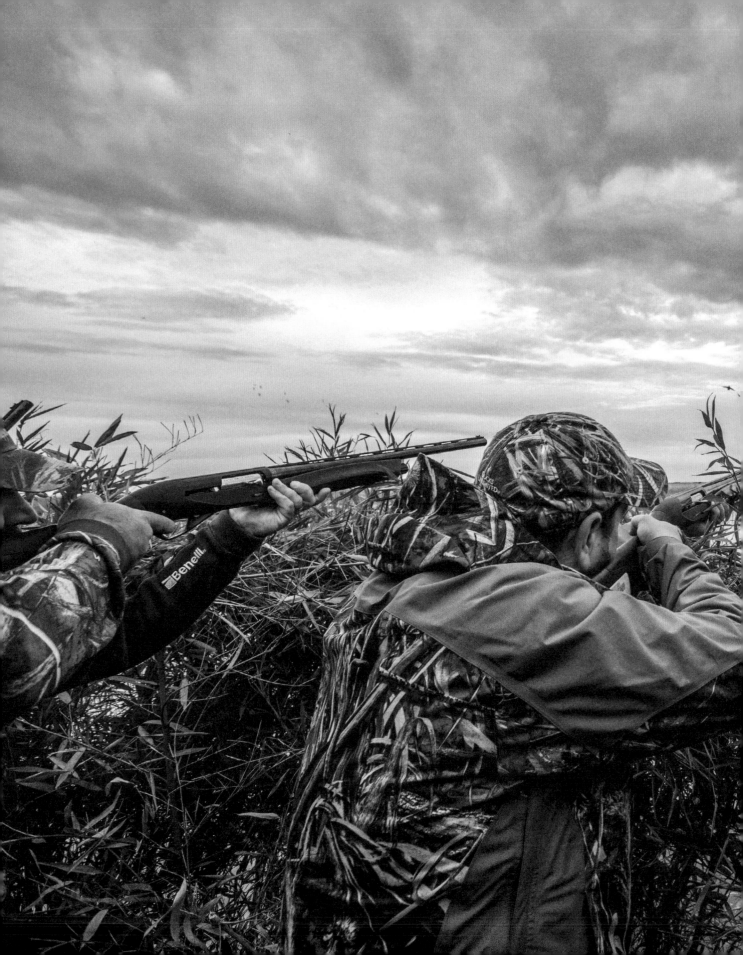

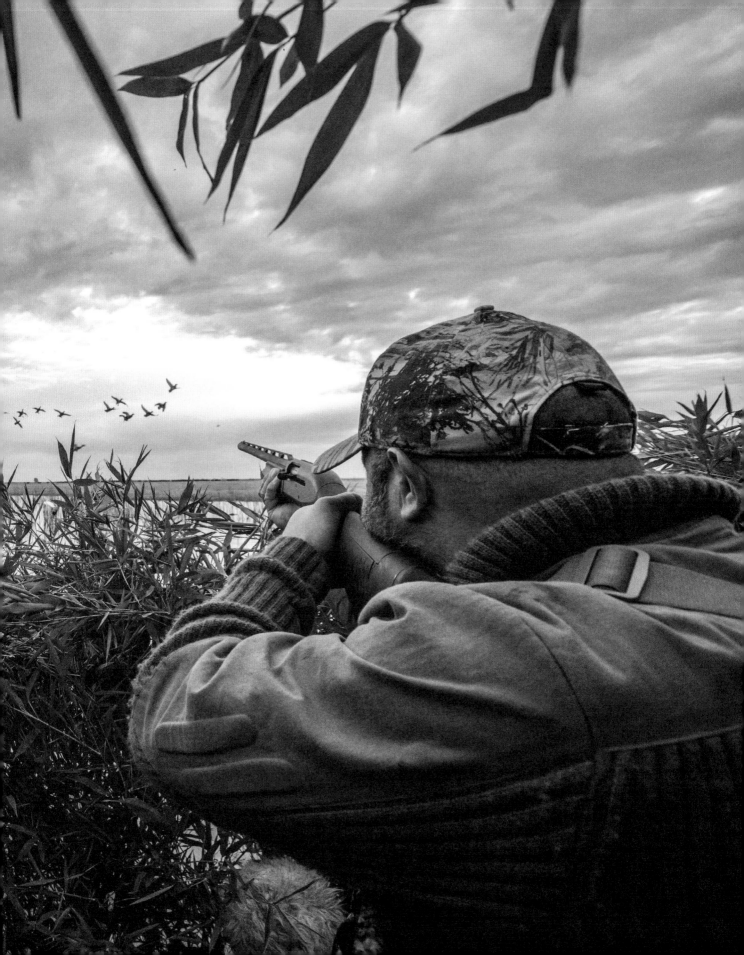

There's a First Time for Everything

Chad Belding

Sometimes it doesn't take much to get the blood flowing. In many cases, it's the little things that count. The very first for anything is special when it comes to positive experiences!

Jim, John, Todd, and Uncle Mel invited me on my first duck hunt. I was curious: They loved it and I wanted to figure out why . . . and that didn't take long. The entire month planning before the hunt was so exciting! I could hear it in their voices. I saw it daily as we put tents, firewood, guns, and ammo into piles ready to be loaded into pickup trucks and trailers to make the voyage to the Sleeper Mine.

The others talked about Sleeper Mine as though it were an X on a treasure map. It was a secret, a duck hunter's desert dreamland. There, the excess runoff water from a gold mine would find its way to the sagebrush flats, where the birds could find sage seeds and weed grass—a buffet of nature's finest crops. Through my binoculars I saw thousands of ducks of all species fall out of the sky with reckless abandon and then swim and eat all their hearts desired. Jim pointed out each species and how to correctly

identify it. See, there are many regulations on migratory duck hunting, and one of my first priorities was to properly identify them. After two hours of scouting these magnificent birds, I was close to ready.

Then it was time for duck camp. A big fire, steaks on the grill, cold soda in hand, real country music coming out of the speakers, and the guys telling stories wilder than you could ever make up. In this moment, I realized that was exactly where I was meant to be and exactly what I had been missing.

I didn't sleep a wink that night before opening day. I smiled at the stars and visualized those big puddle ducks working our decoy spread. You might think I would have been exhausted when the alarm clock went off, but heck, I didn't even need the alarm—I was wide awake before it sounded off. The waders slid on, and the decoy bags were strapped across our backs like a backpack on the first day of school. Our blind bags were stuffed with ammo and snacks, and the dogs were at our side as we began the trek to the honey hole. I distinctly remember the sound of the splash as we tossed each decoy into its intended position. I was put in charge of building out the duck blind to make sure that all four of us would disappear from the hundreds of eyeballs searching us out from above. The dogs were put in place. Jim said, "Twenty minutes until legal light!" I would say I felt like a kid on Christmas morning, but this excitement was far greater than that.

The flooded sagebrush came alive with the sunrise. Mother Nature opened the gate to the wild duck pen and they came. The ducks kept showing up, flooding the morning sky watching and noticing our decoys. We pulled on the jerk string to shake the water. Then, I heard a sound that would hook me on duck hunting for the rest of my life! Jim made a greeter call, and the ducks came in over our heads. "Let them get out there a little bit," Jim said. Then he hit them with a seven-note cadence that emulated a female mallard duck telling the ducks in the air to turn around and come join the party. The flock of gadwalls did just that! It was magic. "Get ready, boys," Jim whispered. I reached for my gun and waited for the signal. Then, when Jim said with excitement, "Get 'em!" our guns fired in sync as we each picked out a target. The next thing I knew, our black lab, Avery, was swimming back our direction with a mouthful of gadwall duck.

I was in 100 percent. From then on, the course of my life would be determined by ducks. That first memorable hunt was all it took to make duck hunting not just a hobby or fascination, but a career and a lifelong love and passion for everything ducks. I learned about preparation. I learned about conservation and respect for the resource. I learned about friend-ship and about camaraderie. Most importantly I learned I would merely exist in a duck's world!

Now, it's my turn to help someone else exchange a mere curiosity into a lifelong passion—to be the inspiration to help someone else experience *their* first duck hunt. And that's what the Provider life is all about.

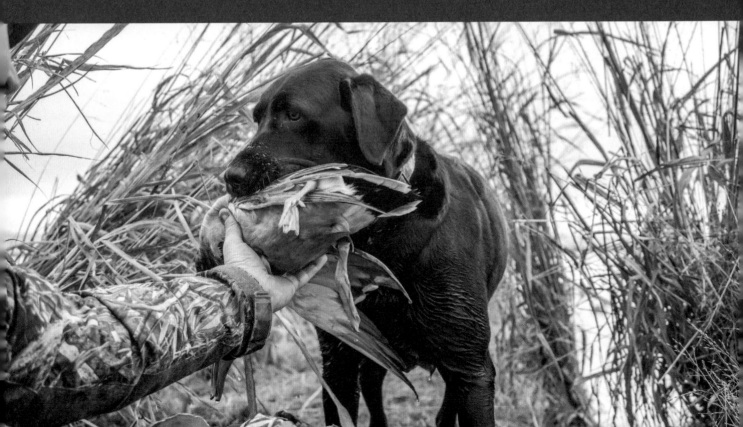

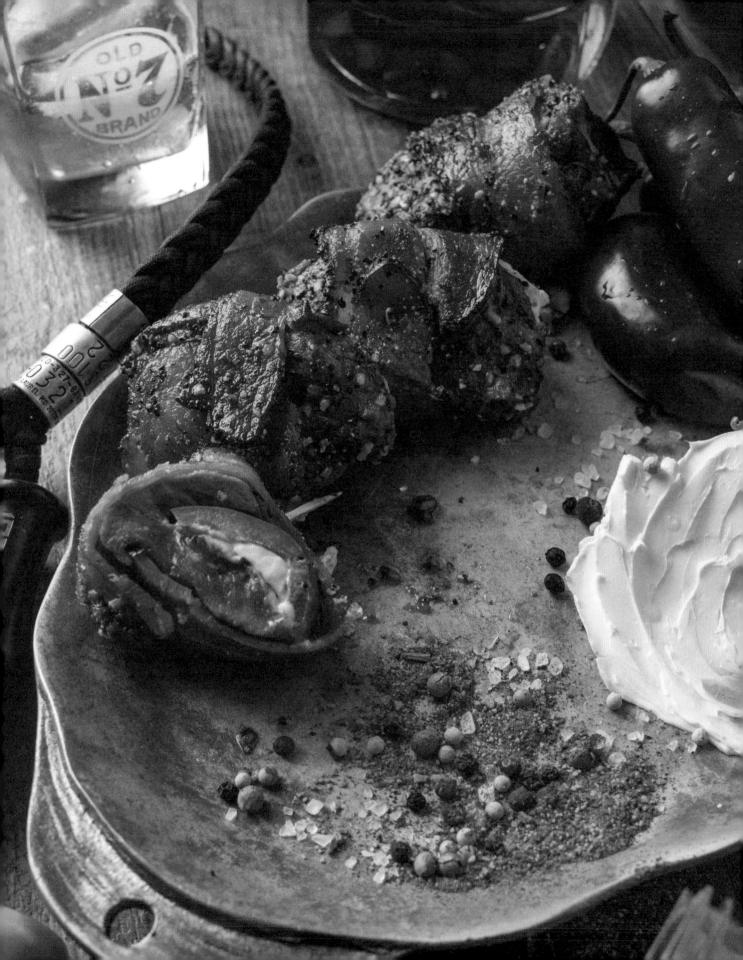

JD's Poppers

SERVES 10–12

This recipe works equally well with ducks and small geese (specks, snows, and lessers).

---

8 boneless, skinless duck or goose breasts

2 cups dry red wine

2 jalapeños, seeded and sliced

3–4 tablespoons cream cheese

8 thin bacon slices

1 tablespoon olive oil

2 tablespoons The Provider Fowl Rub or your favorite spice rub

Garlic powder to taste

Put the breasts in a large bowl, add the wine, cover, and refrigerate for 1 hour.

Preheat your grill (we use a Traeger) to 400°F.

In each breast, cut a deep slit lengthwise on the side that was against the bone to create a pocket. Do not cut all the way through.

Divide the sliced jalapeños evenly among the pockets. Spoon a little cream cheese into each pocket. Wrap each breast tightly with a strip of bacon to close the pocket, then put a toothpick through the whole thing to hold the bacon in place.

Drizzle the olive oil on the stuffed breasts and season with the rub and garlic powder.

Grill the stuffed breasts for 2½–3½ minutes on each side. When you take them off the grill, they will continue to cook for a few minutes; you want them rare to medium-rare so that they do not dry out.

Remove the toothpicks and cut the stuffed breasts in half, if desired.

JD says: "You can choose any type of red wine for this recipe. I use an inexpensive cabernet."

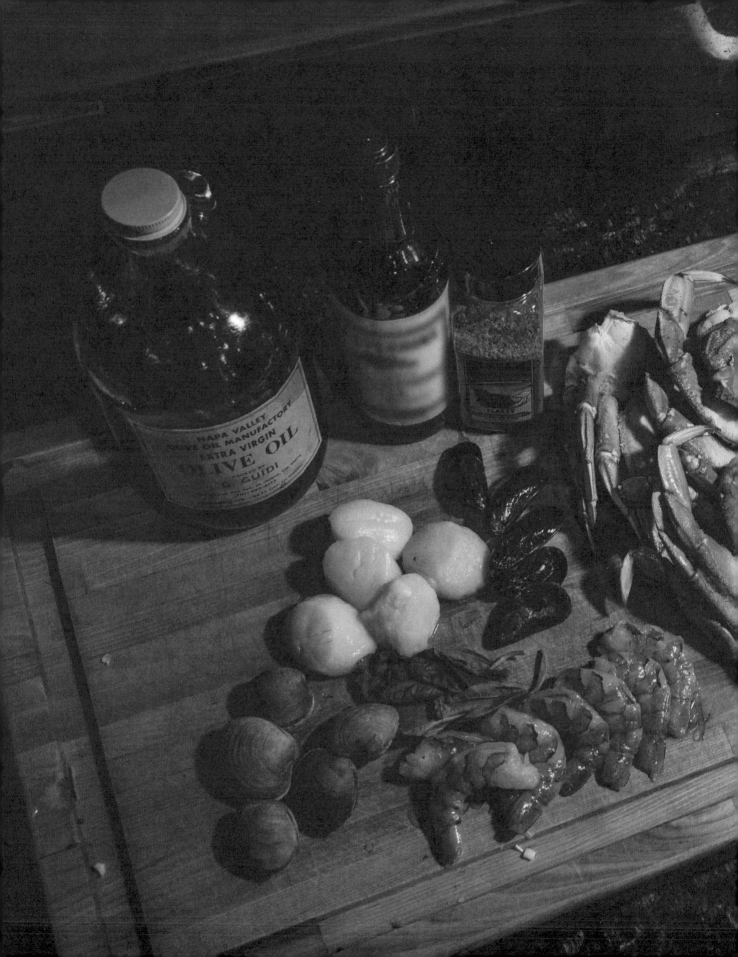

FISH AND SHELLFISH

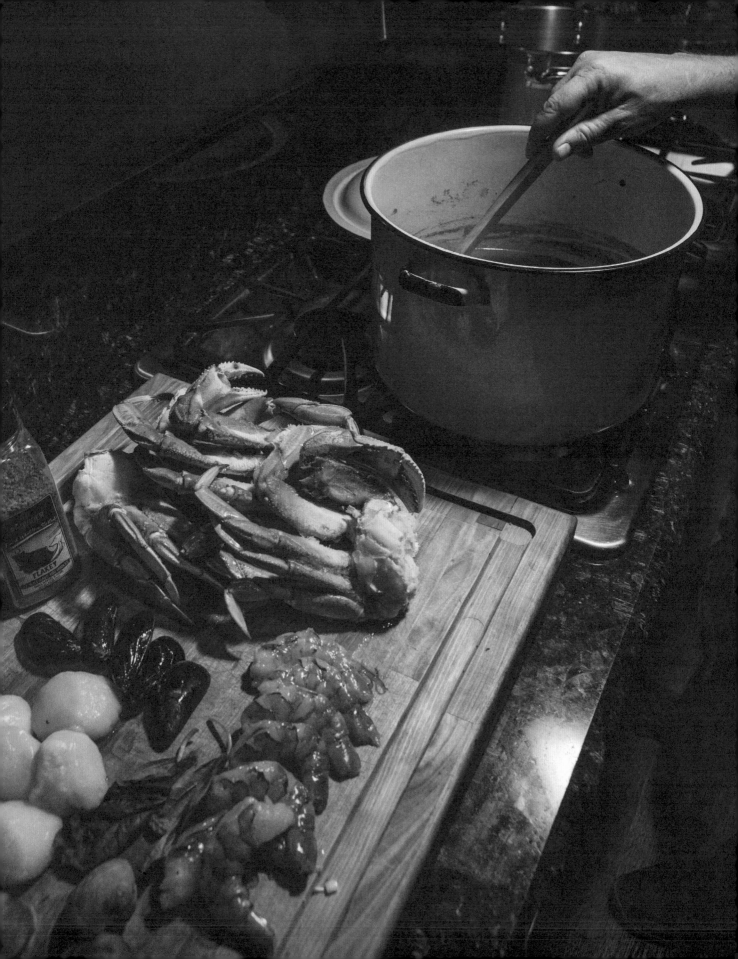

Camping and spending the weekend at the lake was something the Mendes family loved to do. Getting up before the sun, grabbing our fishing gear and walking down to the water's edge was like Christmas Day, each and every time we did it! As we sat there in that cool mountain air, waiting for the lines to start bumping and watching the sun rise over the mountains in front of us, we couldn't help but smile. One of our favorite ways to prepare the fresh fish we would catch was over an open campfire.

Looking back, for Chad Mendes, that feeling was probably the very start of it all—the feeling he would get knowing he had just caught that fish, all on his own, and now he'd enjoy it around a campfire with family, telling fishing stories from the day. That feeling is what being a Provider is all about!

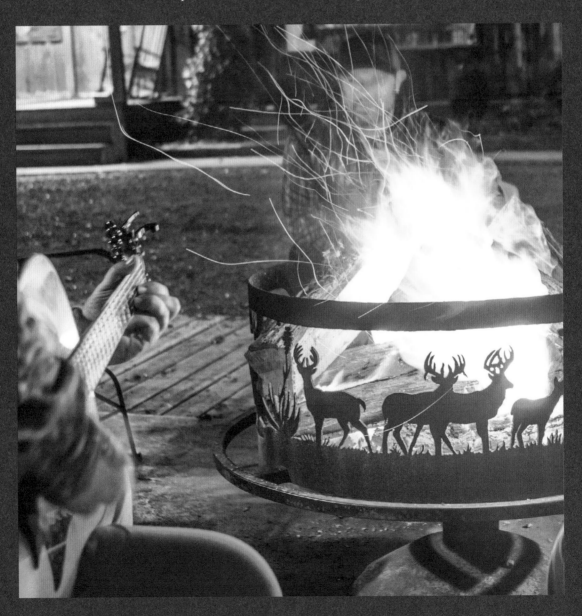

Grammy's Messy Crab

SERVES 4

Chad Belding's assistant, Jennifer Swenson, helped us out a ton with the creation of this cookbook. This is one of her family recipes. She says that messy crab was always on the menu for special occasions. Rich and creamy, this dish made with chunks of freshly cracked crab can be on your table in 30 minutes!

8 tablespoons (1 stick) unsalted butter

2 large onions, chopped

4 garlic cloves, minced

2 tablespoons all-purpose flour

3 cups milk

1 cup whipping cream

2–3 large Dungeness crab legs, cooked, cleaned well, and cracked

Salt and ground black pepper to taste

1 cup chopped fresh parsley

Lemon wedges, for serving

French bread, for serving

In a large saucepan, melt the butter over medium heat. Cook the onions and garlic until the onions are soft, about 5 minutes. Add the flour and cook, stirring, until the flour is golden brown. Remove the pan from the heat and stir in the milk and cream. Return the pan to the heat and bring to a simmer. Stir in the crab. Cover and simmer for 10 minutes, or until heated through. Season with salt and pepper, then stir in the parsley. Ladle the crab and broth into shallow bowls. Serve with lemon wedges and plenty of bread to soak up the sauce.

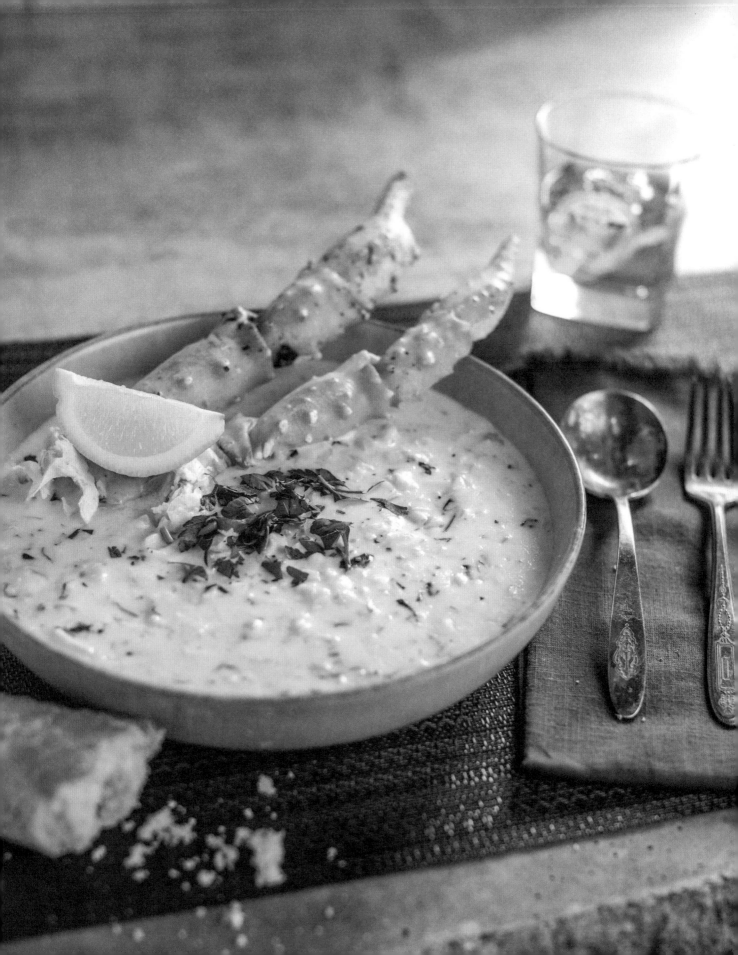

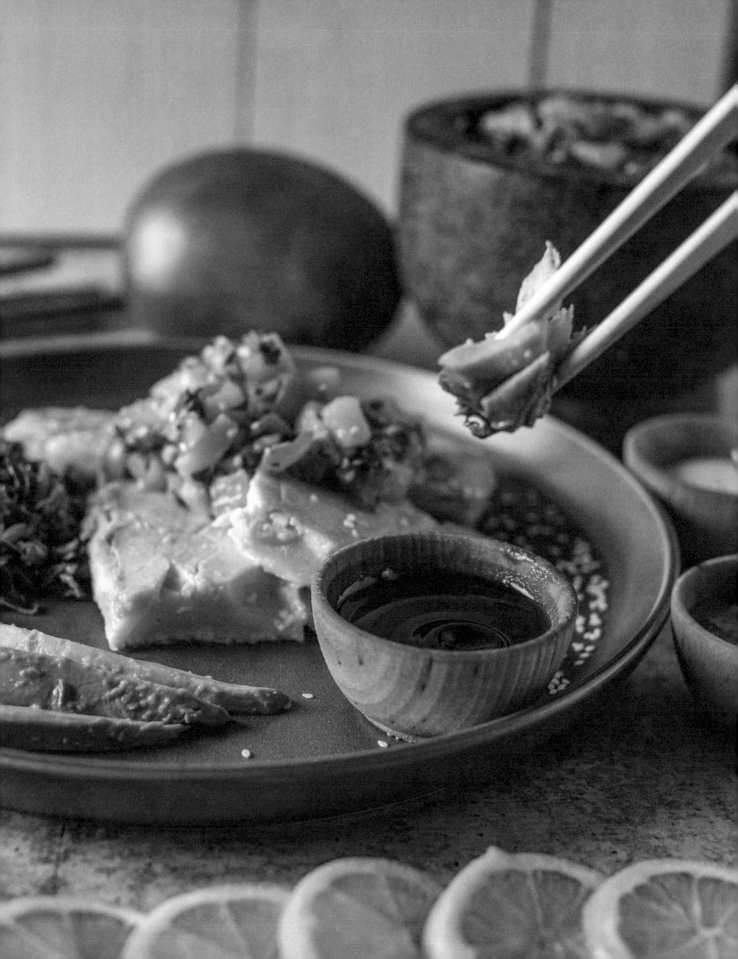

Marinated Yellowtail with Mango Salsa

SERVES 4

This is one of Chad Mendes's favorite fish dishes. If yellowtail isn't available, any white, flaky fish will work. With so many different flavor profiles, this sweet and savory dish will leave you with a smile from ear to ear! It goes great with a nice white wine.

MARINADE

⅓ cup rice wine vinegar

¼ cup olive oil

3 tablespoons toasted sesame oil

1 tablespoon salt

1½ teaspoons garlic power

1½ teaspoons onion powder

1½ teaspoons ground black pepper

2 pounds yellowtail fillets, cut into ½-inch-
   thick pieces

MANGO SALSA

1 mango, peeled, pitted, and cut into small
   cubes

1 avocado, peeled, pitted, and cut into small
   cubes

1 medium tomato, cut into small cubes

1 tablespoon chopped fresh cilantro

1½ teaspoons garlic powder

Salt and ground black pepper to taste

In a large bowl, combine the rice wine vinegar, olive oil, sesame oil, salt, garlic powder, onion powder, and pepper. Add the fish pieces to the bowl and gently toss to coat. Cover and refrigerate for 30 minutes.

While the fish marinates, mix all the salsa ingredients together in a bowl. Cover and refrigerate until you're ready to serve.

Set a cast-iron skillet over high heat or preheat your grill (we use a Traeger) to 450°F. Sear the marinated yellowtail for about 1 minute on each side. This will keep the fish rare in the middle. Remove from the heat and top with mango salsa. Enjoy!

Crab Cakes

MAKES 4-6

We have eaten crab cakes in Seattle and San Francisco and Baltimore, and now we can eat them whenever we want—and we don't live on the coast! Trust us, the flavor of these cakes will make you wonder why you even traveled to those far-off places! For this recipe we like to use our Trinity Oyster Beds, but if you don't have those yet, you can use a baking sheet or cast-iron skillet.

---

1 large egg

¼ cup mayonnaise

15 saltine crackers, crushed, plus more if desired

1 tablespoon chopped fresh parsley

1 teaspoon paprika

1 teaspoon grated lemon zest

1 tablespoon lemon juice

1 teaspoon seasoned salt

¼ teaspoon cayenne pepper

2 dashes hot sauce

1 pound lump blue crab meat, picked over

2 tablespoons Parrain's Cajun Butter (see recipe on page 181), or melted butter

Remoulade sauce, for serving

Sliced green onion, for garnish

Lemon wedges, for serving

In a medium bowl, combine the egg, mayo, crackers, parsley, paprika, lemon zest and juice, seasoned salt, cayenne, and hot sauce and mix well. Add the crab meat and gently toss, being careful not to break up the meat too much. Cover and refrigerate for 30 minutes.

Turn on the broiler on low.

Form the mixture into cakes in the shape of a small egg. Place one in each well of the Trinity Oyster Bed (or place them on a rimmed baking sheet). You can add a few more cracker crumbs to the tops of each cake if you would like a crisp top crust. Lastly, baste each crab cake with Parrain's Cajun Butter. This will aid in creating that nice exterior texture and add a ton of flavor. Broil the crab cakes for about 15 minutes, until lightly browned. Top with a dab of remoulade and garnish with some green onion. Serve with a wedge of lemon and extra remoulade.

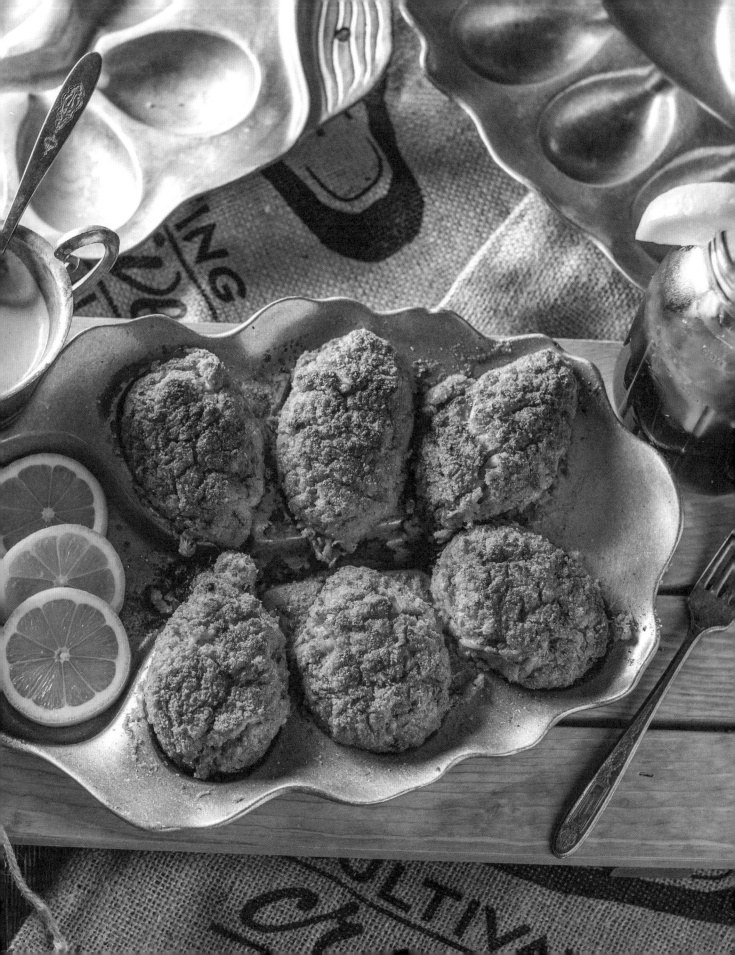

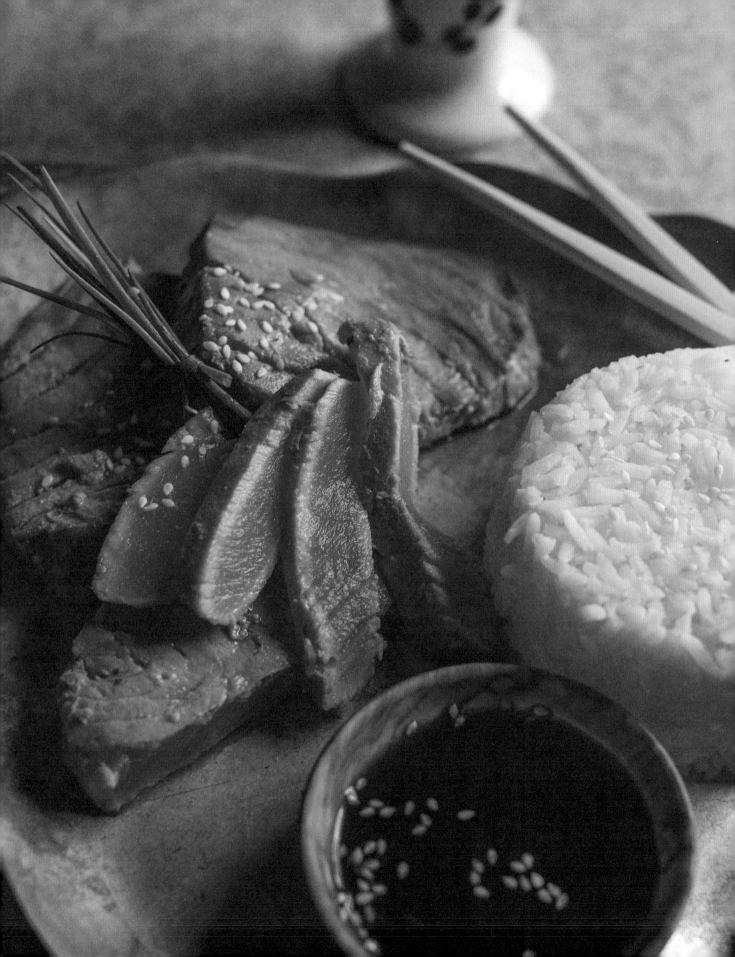

Seared Tuna Medallions

SERVES 4

This quick and easy recipe can be used as an appetizer or served as an entrée alongside your favorite rice and vegetables for an amazing, healthy meal. With East Asian–inspired flavors, you can pair this with your favorite sake or white wine.

¼ cup orange juice

3 tablespoons toasted sesame oil

2 tablespoons rice vinegar

1 tablespoon Worcestershire sauce

1 tablespoon yellow mustard

2 garlic cloves, minced

1 tablespoon sesame seeds

1 (1-pound) tuna steak, cut into ½-inch-thick medallions

In a large resealable plastic bag, mix the orange juice, sesame oil, rice vinegar, Worcestershire, mustard, garlic, and sesame seeds. Add the tuna slices to the marinade, seal, and refrigerate for 1 hour.

Heat a cast-iron skillet over high heat for 5 minutes.

Meanwhile, pour the marinade into a small saucepan, reserving the tuna. Bring the liquid to a boil over medium heat.

Add the tuna medallions to the skillet (there should be a strong sizzle) and sear for 1–2 minutes on each side, depending on how rare you want them. Serve immediately, with the sauce.

West Coast Fish Tacos

MAKES 5 TACOS

Mixing the sweetness of the fruit, the savory flavors of the parmesan cheese, and the kick from the jalapeños yields one of the best fish tacos you will ever taste!

¼ cup olive oil

¼ cup orange juice

Juice of 1 lime

1 tablespoon toasted sesame oil

1 garlic clove, minced

1 teaspoon salt

1 teaspoon ground black pepper

8 ounces yellowtail or any other white, flaky fish fillets

MANDARIN SLAW

1 cup shredded cabbage

⅓ cup chopped pickled carrots

⅓ cup chopped pickled jalapeños

3 mandarin oranges, peeled, sectioned, and each section halved

1 garlic clove, minced

2 tablespoons rice vinegar

1 tablespoon toasted sesame oil

Salt and ground black pepper to taste

TACOS

2 tablespoons olive oil

5 small white corn tortillas

½ cup grated parmesan cheese

Lime wedges

Preheat your grill (we use a Traeger) to 400°F.

In a large bowl, combine the olive oil, orange juice, lime juice, sesame oil, garlic, salt, and pepper and mix well. Add the fish, cover, and refrigerate for 15 minutes.

Meanwhile, in a medium bowl, combine the cabbage, pickled carrots, jalapeños, oranges, garlic, rice vinegar, sesame oil, and a pinch each of salt and pepper. Toss to combine, then cover and refrigerate until you're ready to serve.

Remove the fish from the marinade and grill until firm to the touch, about 7–10 minutes (don't flip). Remove the fish from the grill and cut into chunks.

In a skillet, heat a few drops of olive oil over medium-high heat. Using a circular motion, rub both sides of a tortilla in the oil. Sprinkle a few teaspoons of the parmesan cheese on one side of the tortilla and flip that side down in the pan. Heat for about a minute to melt the cheese, then remove (the cheese side will be the outside of the taco). Repeat with the remaining olive oil, tortillas, and cheese. To make the tacos, add the desired amount of fish, slaw, and a squeeze of lime to each tortilla, fold up, and enjoy!

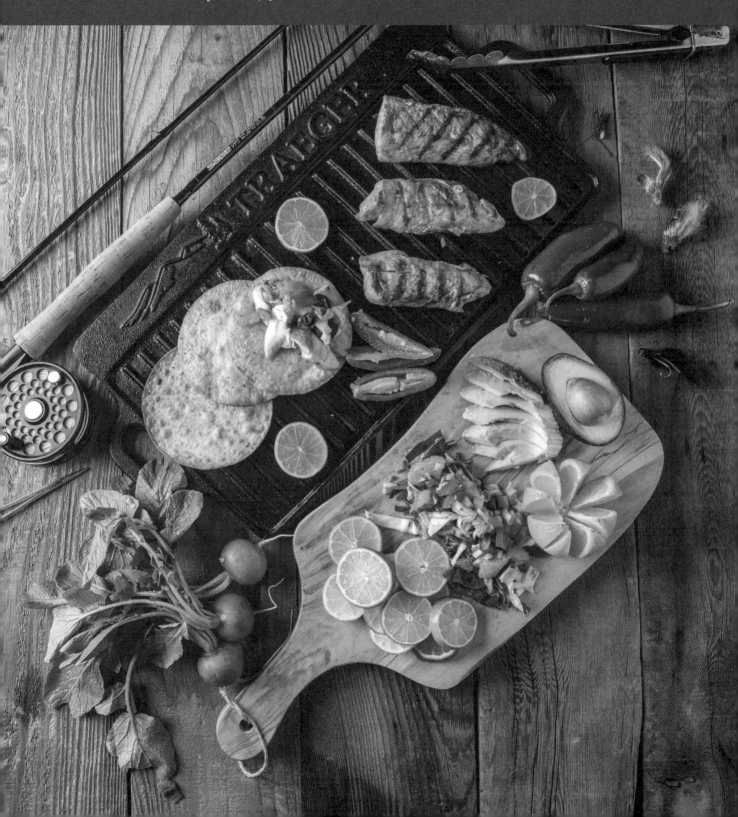

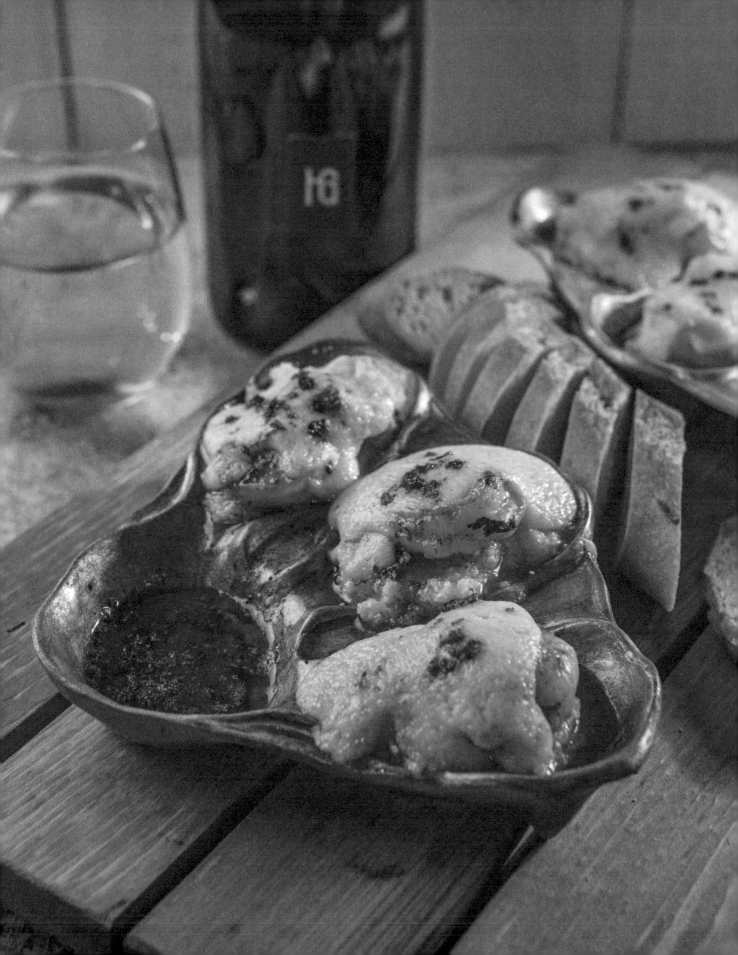

Parrain's Shrimp and Grits with Pepper Jack Cream Sauce

SERVES 4

We have been fortunate enough to visit the South, and that is where we were introduced to shrimp and grits. We have enjoyed this dish in Nashville and in Atlanta and in New Orleans . . . and now in our own backyards on the West Coast! With the help of our friends at the Oyster Bed, we now have the confidence to serve not only perfectly cooked shrimp to our friends and family, but also the most flavorful grits known to man. If you don't have an Oyster Bed yet, use a cast-iron skillet.

2 cups heavy cream

¾ cup all-purpose flour

6 slices pepper Jack cheese

1 pound large white shrimp, peeled and deveined

½ cup Parrain's Cajun Butter (recipe follows) or other compound butter

4 cups cooked grits

½ cup chopped cooked bacon

½ cup chopped green onion

Preheat the oven to 350°F. In a medium saucepan, heat the cream over medium heat. Slowly whisk in the flour until there are no lumps. Lower the heat and add the pepper Jack cheese. Stir until melted and smooth.

Place 2–4 shrimp in each well of an Oyster Bed (or put all of them in a cast-iron skillet) and top with the Cajun butter. Bake for 8 minutes.

Fill each reservoir with grits. Top with the pepper Jack cream sauce, bacon, and green onions and serve.

Parrain's Cajun Butter

¼ cup Parrain's Cajun Butter Seasoning

¼ cup beer or water

2 sticks salted butter, softened

Mix the seasoning and beer to rehydrate the spices. Combine with the softened butter. Refrigerate until ready to use.

Cajun Fried Catfish Sandwiches

SERVES 4

Fried catfish is an icon of Southern cooking. For many, there simply isn't any other way to prepare it. There's something about a cornmeal crust that goes perfectly with the catfish. We aren't sure who decided to fry a catfish in the first place, but one thing is for sure: we are really glad they decided not to keep it a secret. Get you a bun and an appetite, because you won't be able to stop at one of these sandwiches.

Nonstick cooking spray

⅔ cup yellow cornmeal

¼ cup all-purpose flour

1½ teaspoons seasoned salt

½ teaspoon ground black pepper

½ teaspoon cayenne pepper

½ teaspoon lemon pepper

¼ teaspoon paprika

2 large eggs

2 teaspoons hot sauce

1 pound fresh catfish fillets

2 cups canola oil

SANDWICHES

Tartar sauce

Hoagie buns, split

Shredded lettuce

Lemon wedges

Hot sauce

Lightly spray a rimmed baking sheet with cooking spray.

In a brown paper bag, combine the cornmeal, flour, seasoned salt, black pepper, cayenne, lemon pepper, and paprika and shake together.

In a deep pie plate, whisk together the eggs and hot sauce.

Dip a catfish fillet into the egg mixture, then add to the bag with the dry ingredients and shake liberally to coat. Place the fillet on the greased baking sheet. Repeat with each fillet. Put the baking sheet in the refrigerator for 15 minutes.

Heat the canola oil in a large Dutch oven or deep fryer to 340°F. Working in batches, gently add the catfish fillets and fry until golden brown on both sides, about 3 minutes total. Do not crowd the fish in the fryer. Transfer to a plate lined with paper towels.

Spread tartar sauce on both sides of each hoagie bun. Place a fillet on one half, then top with some lettuce, a squeeze of lemon, and a couple dashes of your favorite hot sauce. Close the sandwich and dig in!

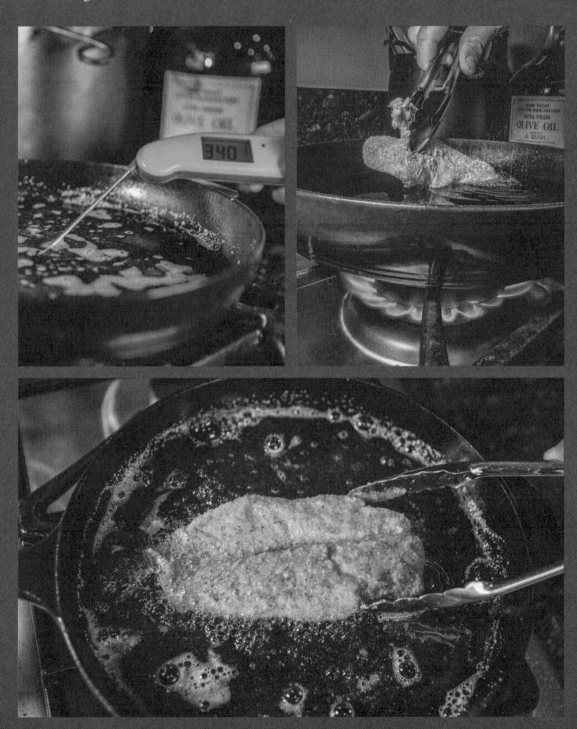

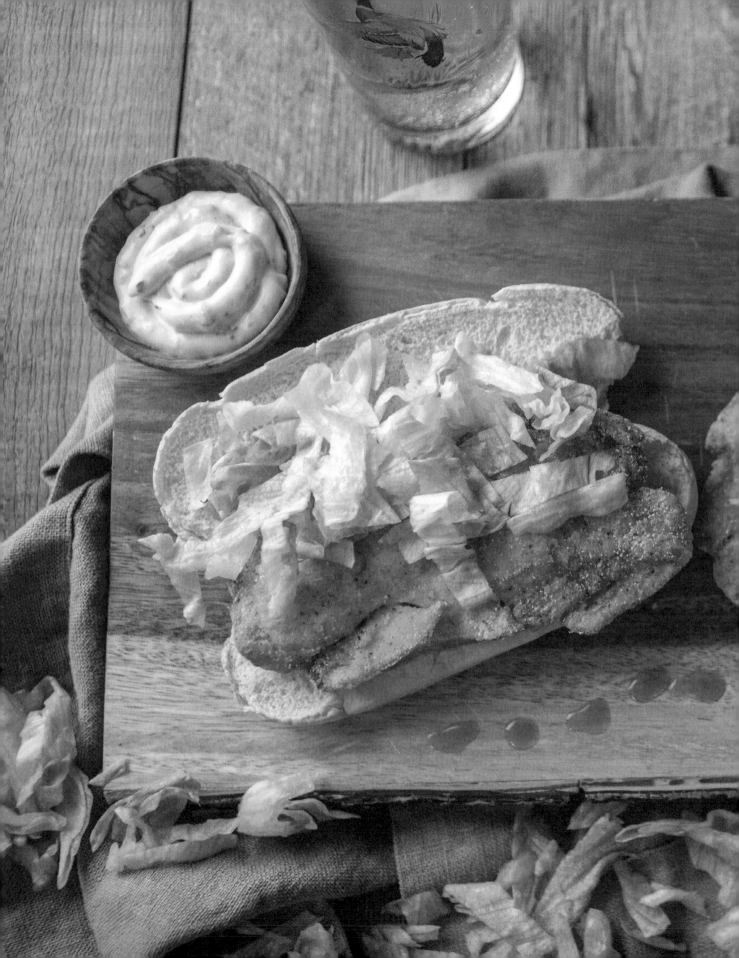

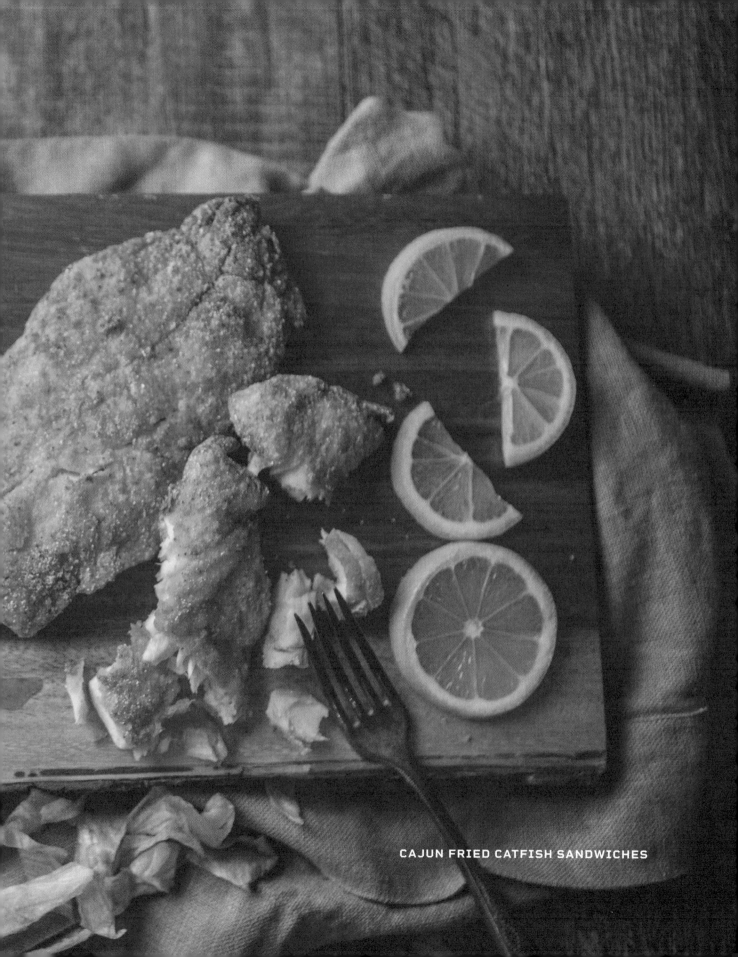

CAJUN FRIED CATFISH SANDWICHES

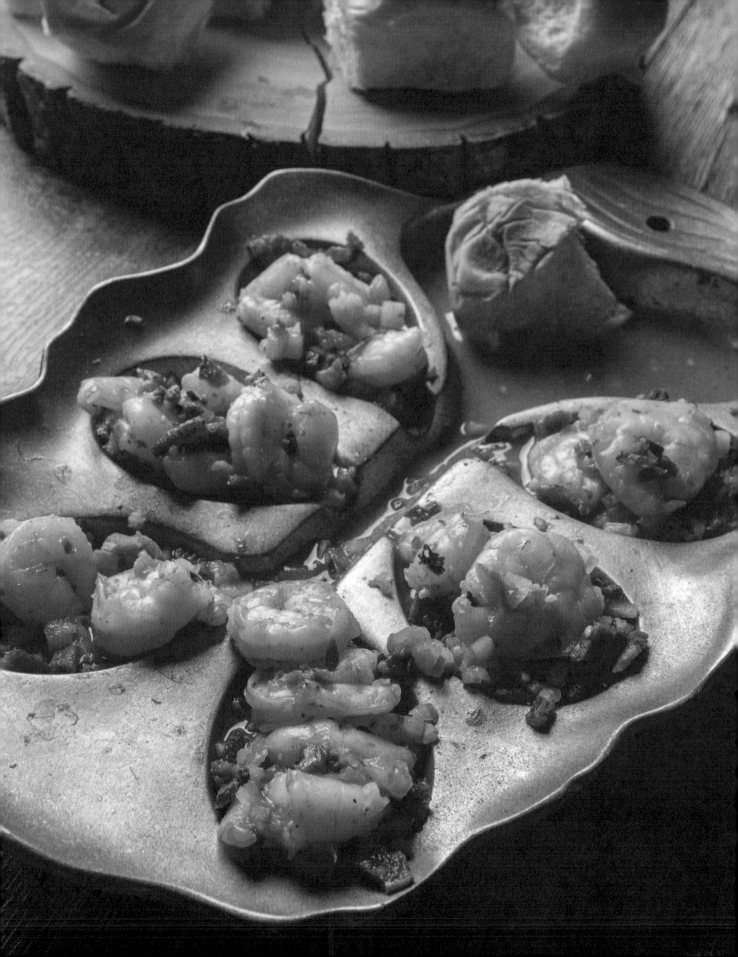

Caribbean Shrimp Appetizer

SERVES 6-8

Oyster Bed is all about flavor—and making it easy! Well, it doesn't get any easier or tastier than this shrimp appetizer. If you don't have an Oyster Bed yet, feel free to use a cast-iron skillet.

---

1 cup finely chopped pineapple

¾ cup finely chopped red onion

½ cup finely chopped red bell pepper

¼ cup chopped fresh cilantro

¾ cup pineapple juice

¾ cup sweet chili sauce

Nonstick cooking spray

3 bacon slices, cooked and finely chopped

2 pounds medium to large shrimp, peeled and deveined

Pickled sliced jalapeños (optional)

12 slider buns, such as King's Hawaiian Original Sweet Rolls

Preheat your grill (we use a Traeger) to 350°F.

In a medium bowl, mix the pineapple, onion, bell pepper, and cilantro.

Mix the pineapple juice and sweet chili sauce in a large measuring cup.

Place two Stella or Le Petite Oyster Beds on the grill. Allow the cookware to heat up for 5 minutes, then spray thoroughly with cooking spray. In each well, drop a small amount of bacon and place two or three shrimp on top. It should be sizzling nicely without burning your bacon. Top the shrimp with 1 tablespoon of the pineapple salsa, 1 tablespoon of the sauce mix, and a little more bacon. If you like it spicy, add a slice of pickled jalapeño. Close the lid and cook for 2–3 minutes.

Remove the Oyster Beds from the heat and place on a trivet. The shrimp should be just a tiny bit underdone when you remove them from the heat because they will continue to cook for a minute or two. Much of the sauce should be rendered down from the wells and into the reservoir. Place the Oyster Bed in the center of your dining table with a serving spoon and a basket of rolls to sop up the sauce. Serve with extra pineapple salsa alongside.

Yellowtail Poke

SERVES 4–5

Chad Mendes's great friend Ryan originally introduced us to this dish. Ryan is a huge offshore fisherman and always has fresh tuna and yellowtail in his freezer. You can't go wrong sitting on the beach with a beer in hand, scooping this stuff up with tortilla chips!

1 pound yellowtail fillets, cubed

1 avocado, peeled, pitted, and cubed

¼ cup chopped green onion

2 tablespoons toasted sesame oil

1 tablespoon soy sauce

1 tablespoon toasted sesame seeds

1½ teaspoons garlic powder

Tortilla chips, for serving

In a medium bowl, combine all the ingredients. Toss to combine, cover, and refrigerate for at least 2 hours. Serve with tortilla chips for dipping.

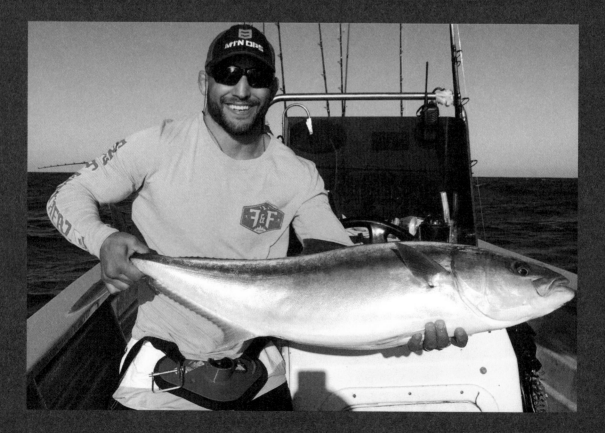

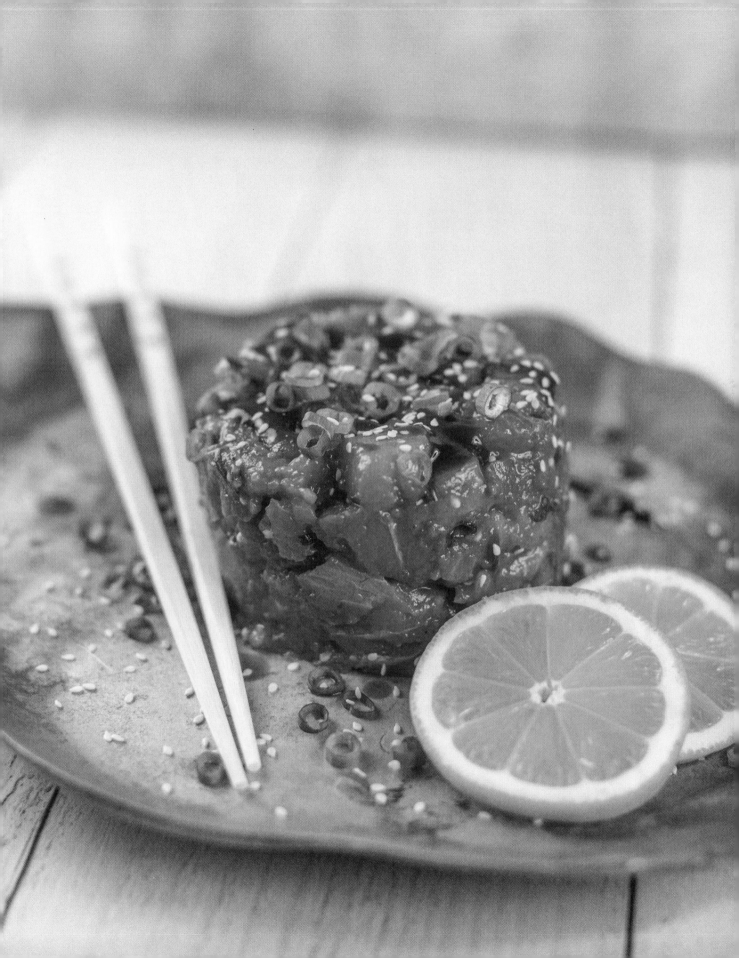

Fitness Tips

Chad Mendes

A Provider needs to be physically ready for the hunt and for whatever life throws their way. Here are some training principles that I followed throughout my career as an athlete; I still use them today to keep my body in top shape.

Start small. The worst thing you can do is jump right into a hard, extreme training session and either injure yourself or get so broken down that you can't do anything for days or weeks after. Build up the intensity of your workouts and set goals to meet along the way. This will keep you motivated and build confidence as you see improvements being made.

Make sure you have proper nutrition. It's crucial to have the right nutrition before, during, and after your workouts. Typically I like a complex carb like whole oats and a lean protein an hour or two before my workout. During my workout, I sip on a scoop (about 20 grams) of whey protein in a simple sugar mixture like Gatorade or even a high-octane carb like Vitargo. Then I make sure to eat a high-calorie meal rich in protein and carbohydrates about an hour after my workout. I notice that this system

helps keep my muscles from tearing down too much during extreme workouts and helps recovery time tremendously. Also, be sure to eat breakfast! Having a lean protein will kick-start your metabolism for the day and get your body out of the "fasting" mode it was in overnight. It's now burning calories, and that's what you want! Remember to eat every three to four hours to keep your metabolism burning along.

Get comfortable being uncomfortable. Gains are made in those moments when you want to quit. This feeling is something I recommend you try and get to know well. You may never become best friends with it, but that's OK! Figuring out what it takes to keep your body and mind pushing forward during those uncomfortable times will strengthen you both inside and outside the gym.

Don't stress if you hit a plateau. This is very common, even among world-class athletes. Small things can be adjusted or tweaked to start climbing again. If it's weight-related, it might be as simple as adding another mile or two when you exercise or adjusting your calorie intake. This can be done over each meal throughout the day so it's not a big reduction in calories from one meal.

RECOVER. RECOVER. RECOVER. It took me quite a few years into my athletic career to learn that recovery is just as important as training! It doesn't matter if you train harder than anyone in the world; if you are overtrained and run down, you will never be at your best. So many times my ten-week training camp for a fight would be three extremely hard MMA training sessions a day, six or seven days a week. By week eight I felt so run down I would get sick, feel weak and flat, and usually feel worse going into a fight than when I started my camp. I soon learned I needed to set aside time to recover. It's definitely a fine line between taking too much time off and not enough, but you need to figure out what that amount of rest time is. Everyone's different, so it will vary from person to person. Sauna stretching, cryotherapy, massages, light runs or bike rides, and light swimming are all things I would do for recovery during my training. The most important key to recovery, though, is enough sleep! Make sure you are getting at least eight hours of sleep each night. I recommend making this a priority.

Visualize success. Seeing yourself stepping on that scale and reaching your goal. Seeing yourself scoring that winning point in the last few seconds. Seeing yourself getting a KO to win a big fight. Seeing yourself making that stalk on a giant bull elk and executing the shot perfectly. Visualizing yourself being successful is not only very motivating, it's also a great way to train your mind into doing what you want it to in those moments when you don't have time to sit and think and you just react. If you truly believe something and decide to do the work necessary, chances are you are going to be successful. This saying has always stuck with me: "The harder you work, the luckier you get."

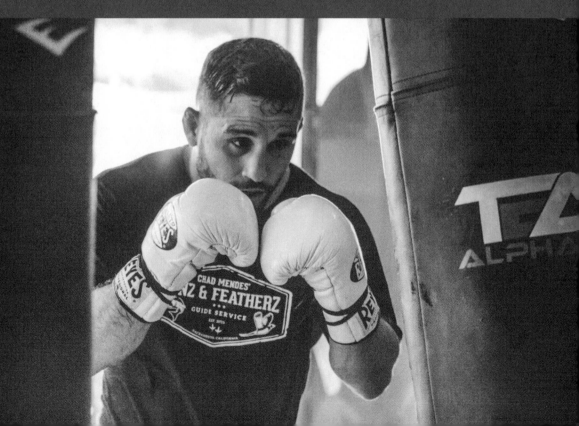

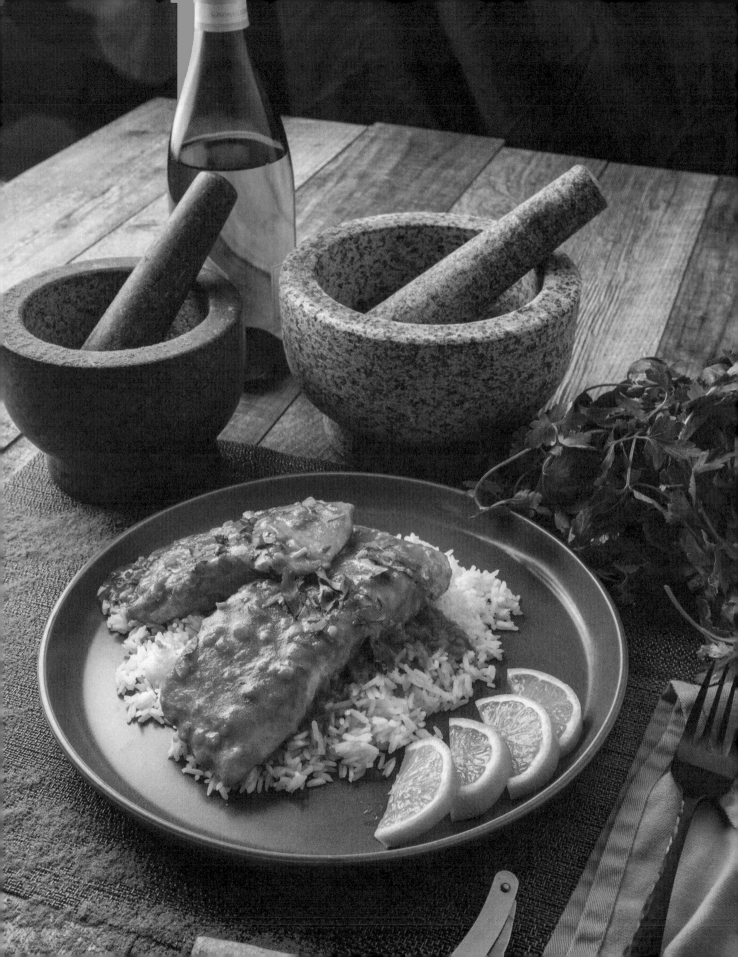

Brian's Coconut Curry Halibut

SERVES 4

Chad Mendes's good buddy Brian has lived on the northern coast of California his entire life. Seafood is his jam! This dish is a beautiful addition to your fish recipes and will pair amazingly well with a good buttery Chardonnay.

---

3 tablespoons coconut oil, divided

1–2 skinless halibut fillets

½ sweet onion, diced

3 garlic cloves, minced

1 tablespoon peeled and finely minced ginger

3 teaspoons yellow curry powder, divided

2 teaspoons ground coriander

¼ cup yellow curry paste

1 (13.6-ounce) can full-fat coconut milk

1½ cups chicken stock

½ teaspoon cornstarch mixed with ¼ cup water (optional)

¼ cup chopped fresh cilantro

1 tablespoon lemon juice

2 teaspoons fish sauce

2 teaspoons sugar

Salt and ground black pepper to taste

Steamed rice, for serving

In a large, deep skillet, heat 1 tablespoon of the coconut oil over medium-high heat. Quickly sear both sides of the halibut fillets; the fish will still be raw in the middle. Transfer the fillets to a plate.

Add the remaining 2 tablespoons coconut oil to the skillet and heat over medium-high heat. Add the onion and cook until tender, about 5 minutes. Add the garlic and ginger and cook for about 2 minutes, until fragrant. Reduce the heat to low and add 2 teaspoons of the curry powder, the coriander, and the curry paste. Stir well and cook for about 2 minutes, until lightly toasted. Pour in the coconut milk and chicken stock. With a wooden spoon, scrape the bottom of the skillet to incorporate any cooked-on pieces of fish and onion. Bring everything to a rapid simmer and cook, stirring occasionally, for 20–30 minutes, until the sauce is the desired thickness. If your sauce is still looking thin, stir in the cornstarch slurry. Add the cilantro, lemon juice, fish sauce, and sugar and stir.

Return the halibut fillets to the skillet and simmer in the sauce for 5–10 minutes, until the fish has reached the desired doneness. Season with salt and pepper. Serve the halibut fillets over a bed of rice and sprinkle with the remaining 1 teaspoon curry powder.

Cioppino

SERVES 6-8

This seafood stew originated in San Francisco in the late 1800s. We have heard many stories on how it got its name. Our favorite story is that it was created by fishermen living in the North Beach area of the city. When these Italian immigrant fishermen returned from a day on the boats, they would gather around and "chip in" a portion of the day's catch to the stew. This often consisted of fish, clams, squid, and shrimp. In their heavy accents, "chip in" morphed into "cioppino," and a legendary seafood stew was born. Serve this version, courtesy of our friend Jim Rhea, with some sourdough garlic bread.

SAUCE

½ cup olive oil

2 medium onions, chopped

4 garlic cloves, chopped

½ cup chopped fresh parsley

¼ cup chopped fresh basil

1½ tablespoons sugar

1 tablespoon celery salt

Dash Worcestershire sauce

1 (28-ounce) can crushed tomatoes

3½ cups water (fill the empty tomato can!)

3 bay leaves

Pinch crushed red pepper

Pinch ground cinnamon

SEAFOOD

¼ cup olive oil

2 tablespoons unsalted butter

3 garlic cloves, chopped

12 ounces littleneck clams

½ cup sliced fennel

½ cup dry white wine (or more)

8 ounces mussels

8 ounces cleaned squid

Pinch saffron

2 pounds cracked cooked Dungeness crab

12 ounces large scallops

12 ounces cod or other firm white fish, cut into bite-size pieces

12 ounces large shrimp, peeled and deveined

In a large saucepan, heat the olive oil over medium heat. Add the onions, garlic, parsley, and basil and cook until the onions are translucent but not brown. Stir in the sugar, celery salt, and Worcestershire. Add the tomatoes, water, bay leaves, crushed red pepper, and cinnamon, reduce the heat, and let simmer for 1 hour. (The sauce can be made up to 2 days ahead of time; cover and refrigerate, then bring back to a simmer before proceeding).

In a large pot with a lid, heat the olive oil, butter, and garlic over medium-high heat. Throw in the clams and fennel and steam for 3–5 minutes, until the clams open. Add the white wine, mussels, squid, and saffron. Steam until the mussels open, about 5 minutes. Add the simmering sauce and stir gently. Add the crab, scallops, cod, and shrimp and cook for 20 minutes. (Do not stir too much or it will break up the white fish.) Remove and discard the bay leaves, as well as any clams or mussels that did not open. Ladle the stew into shallow bowls and serve with plenty of bread for sopping up the sauce.

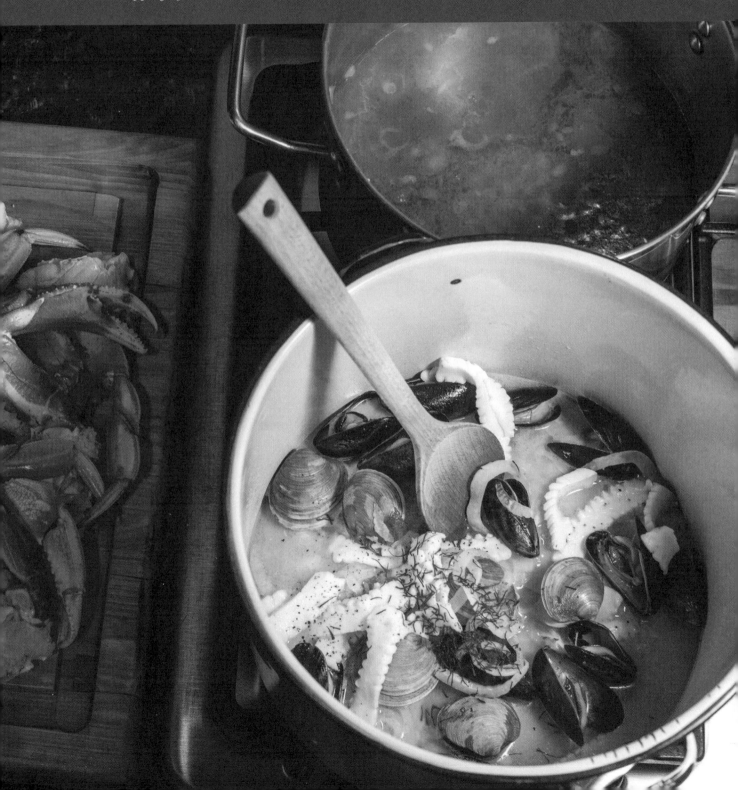

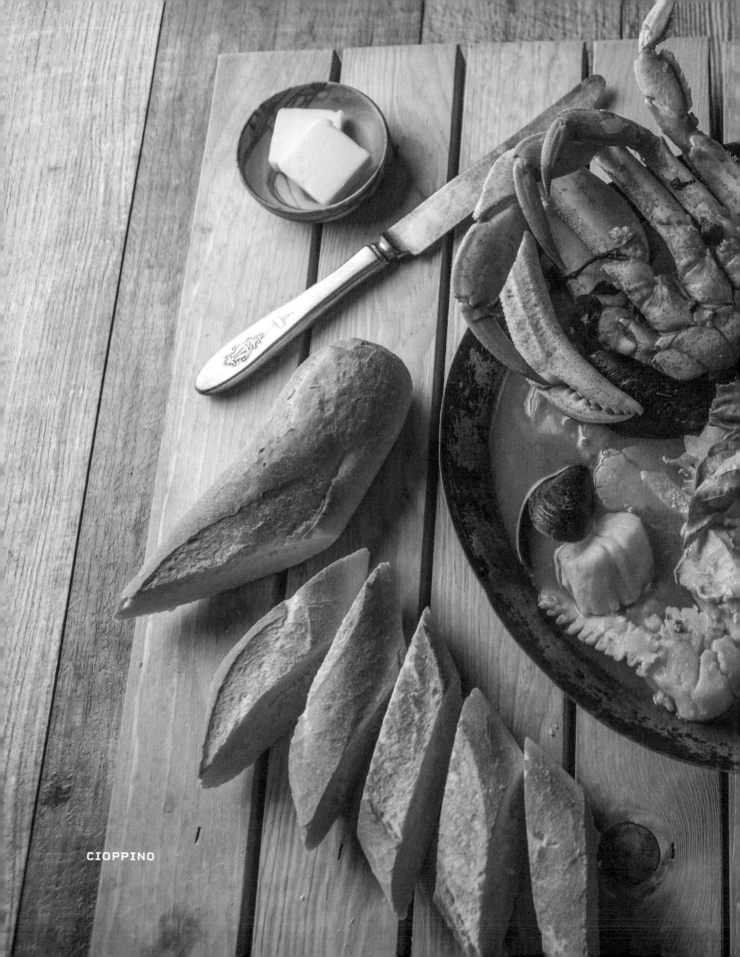

CIOPPINO

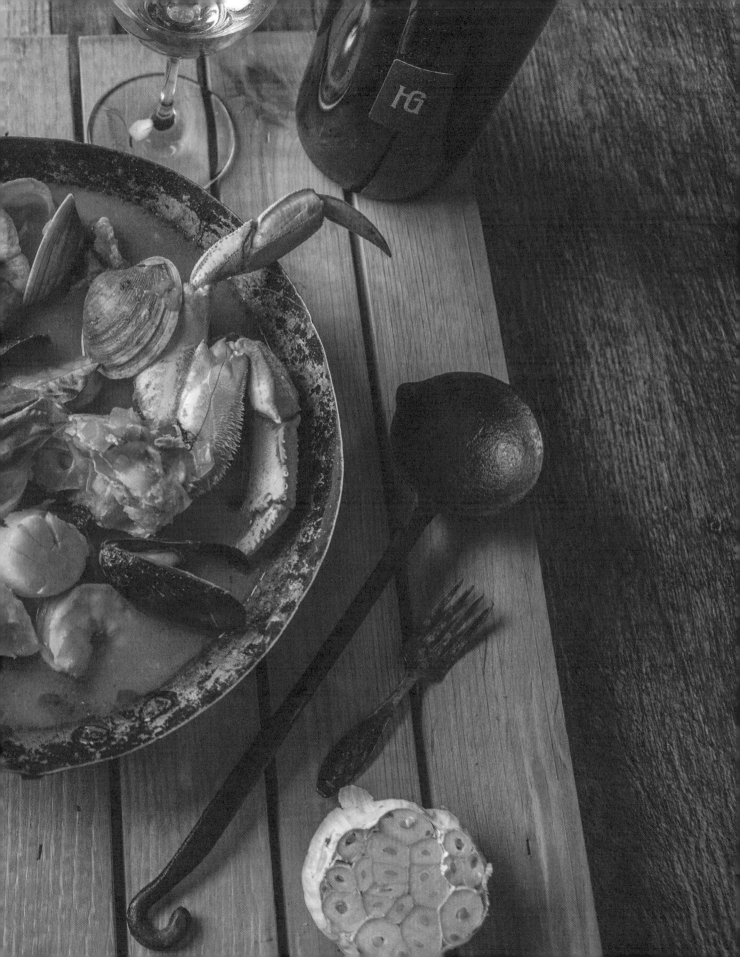

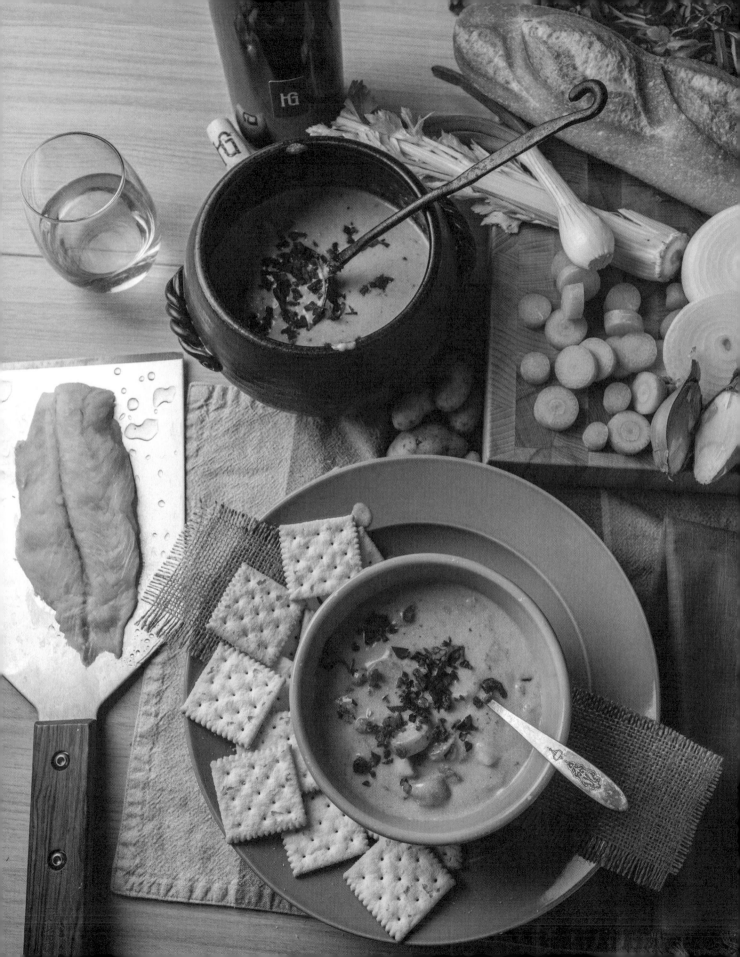

Brad's Killer Striper Chowder

SERVES 6-8

Our buddy Brad Forsythe is a master Provider! He hunts. He gardens. And he fishes. And when he fishes, he's all about that striper chowdah! He came up with this variation from many experiences with that famous Boston dish, and he added one of the tastiest fishes in North America. Enjoy it, you pirates!

---

8 tablespoons (1 stick) unsalted butter, divided

1 white onion, diced

½ shallot, diced

2 celery stalks, diced

1 carrot, peeled and diced

1 thyme sprig, stemmed and chopped

4 cups clam juice or fish stock, divided

2–3 Yukon Gold potatoes, finely chopped

6 pepper bacon slices

5 tablespoons all-purpose flour

1 quart half-and-half

12 ounces fresh-caught striped bass fillets, cut into cubes

1 quart heavy whipping cream

Salt and ground black pepper to taste

Fresh parsley, for garnish

In a stockpot, melt 4 tablespoons (½ stick) of the butter over medium heat. Add the onion, shallot, celery, carrot, and thyme and cook until the onion is translucent, about 3 minutes.

Add 3 cups of the clam juice and the potatoes (the small pieces will dissolve and thicken the chowder). Boil for 40 minutes.

Meanwhile, in a medium skillet, cook the bacon over medium-high heat until fully cooked, about 6 minutes. Transfer the bacon to a plate lined with paper towels, reserving the drippings in the skillet. When cool enough to handle, chop up the cooked bacon.

Add the remaining 4 tablespoons (½ stick) butter to the skillet with the bacon drippings. Whisk in the flour to form a roux, about 2 minutes. Add the remaining 1 cup clam juice and whisk until smooth. Stir in the half-and-half and about one-third of the striper meat. Reduce the heat and simmer for 30 minutes.

Stir the roux mixture and the cream into the potato chowder base, stirring frequently to get the desired consistency. Simmer for 10 minutes, then add the bacon and remaining striper meat. Simmer for 5 minutes. Season with salt and pepper, garnish with a little fresh parsley, and serve!

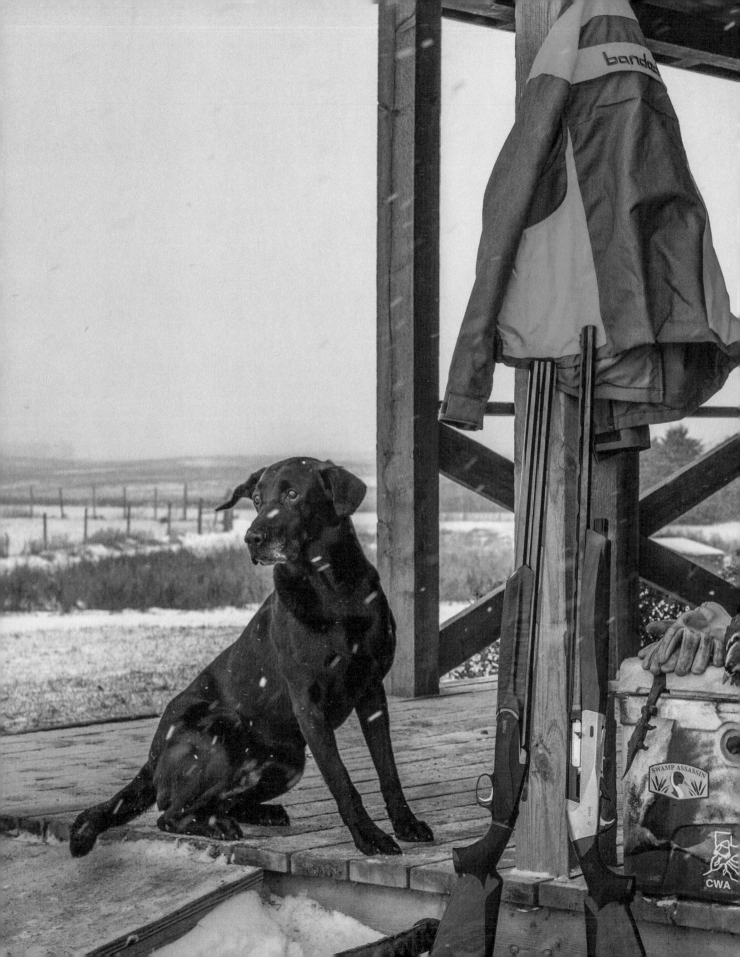

DOMESTIC MEATS

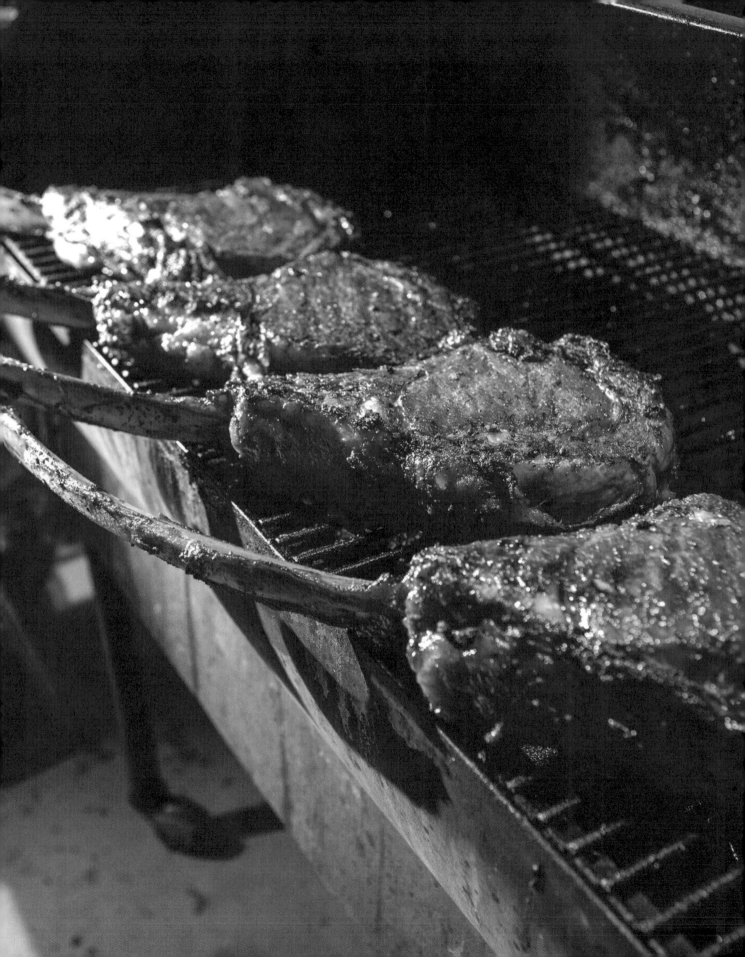

Whether you prefer lump coal, charcoal briquettes, gas, or pellets, we can all agree that life is better when we gather around a grill. Your love for the grill may have begun when you were young and watched your dad char a steak with a beer in one hand and tongs clicking in the other—it just does not get any cooler than that! Or maybe it was your college days, standing in the parking lot of the stadium grilling hot dogs and waiting to scream for your team. Your love for grilling followed all the way to buying your first house and clumsily putting together your first brand-new grill, and grilled meats have been with you through thick and thin.

Let's face it, no one goes to the beach with a slow cooker! We do not have backyard quiche parties. Standing in front of a hot grill and putting your spin on age-old recipes for friends and family is a relatable experience to almost everyone. People in the frozen north can be found around a grill on the coldest of nights, just as the sweat rolls off your favorite southern pit master. I suppose what we are trying to say is there is a common bond felt with all those who grill. Much like those who hunt, fish, or play sports, the specifics can be argued, but the common denominator will always be respected!

These recipes, based on conventional proteins like beef, pork, and chicken, will give you many reasons to fire up your beloved grill or smoker. You'll also find some delicious soups and stews for those colder nights, too.

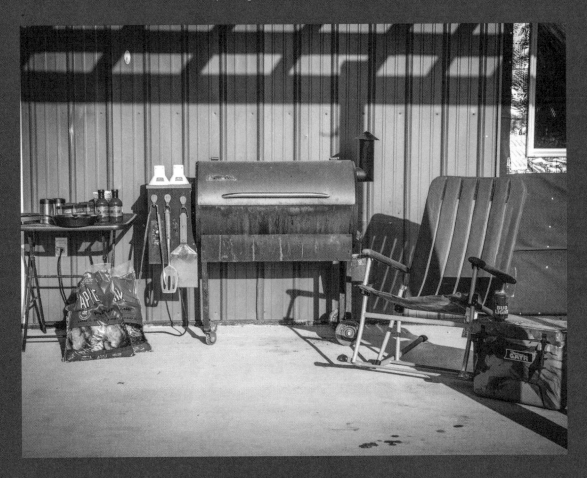

Candied Pork Chops

SERVES 6

We hunt wild boar and we raise perfect pigs—either way, their chops are going on the table! We never settle when it comes to bringing out the best in our pork offerings, and we feel that this recipe is one for the ages. We could have gone so many routes with a pork chop dish but when the dust settled, the decision was unanimous: This is the champion!

---

2 cups dark brown sugar

1 cup dark soy sauce

1 teaspoon granulated garlic

1 teaspoon ground black pepper

12 thin-cut bone-in pork chops

In a small bowl, combine the brown sugar, soy sauce, garlic, and pepper. Mix well until it forms a paste.

Put the pork chops in a baking dish and cover with the brown sugar mixture. Be sure to get both sides of the pork chops covered in the mixture. Cover with plastic wrap and refrigerate for at least 6 hours—overnight is better.

Set your grill/smoker (we use Traeger) on smoke for 5 minutes, then preheat to 450°F.

Remove the pork chops from the dish and place on the grill grate. Cook for 3–5 minutes per side, until the chops are cooked through and have a dark candied exterior. Serve immediately.

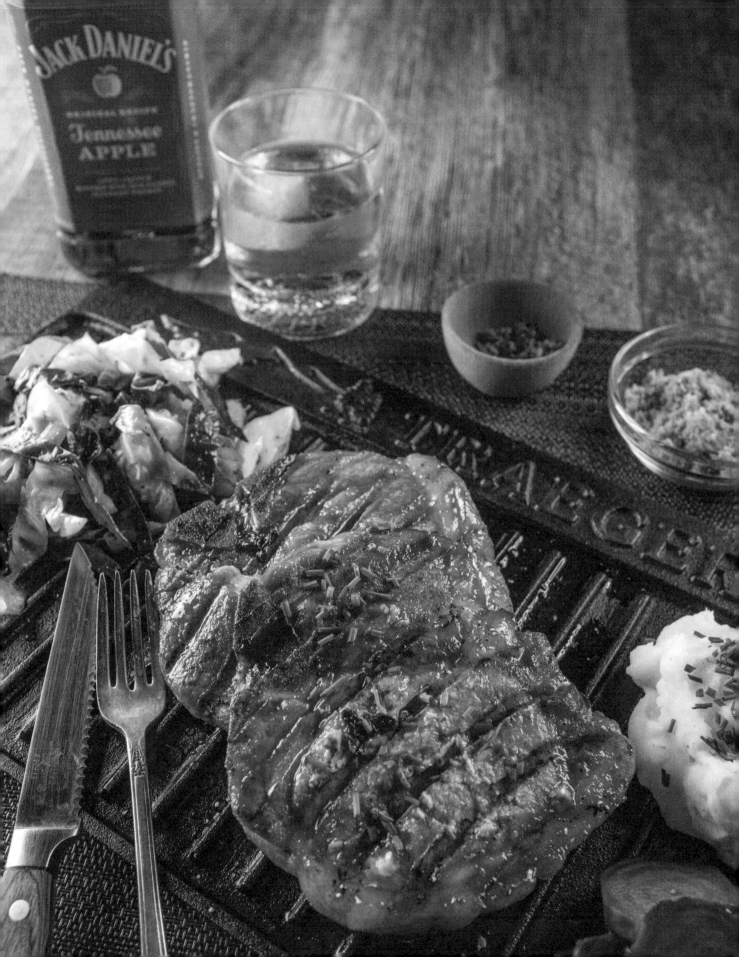

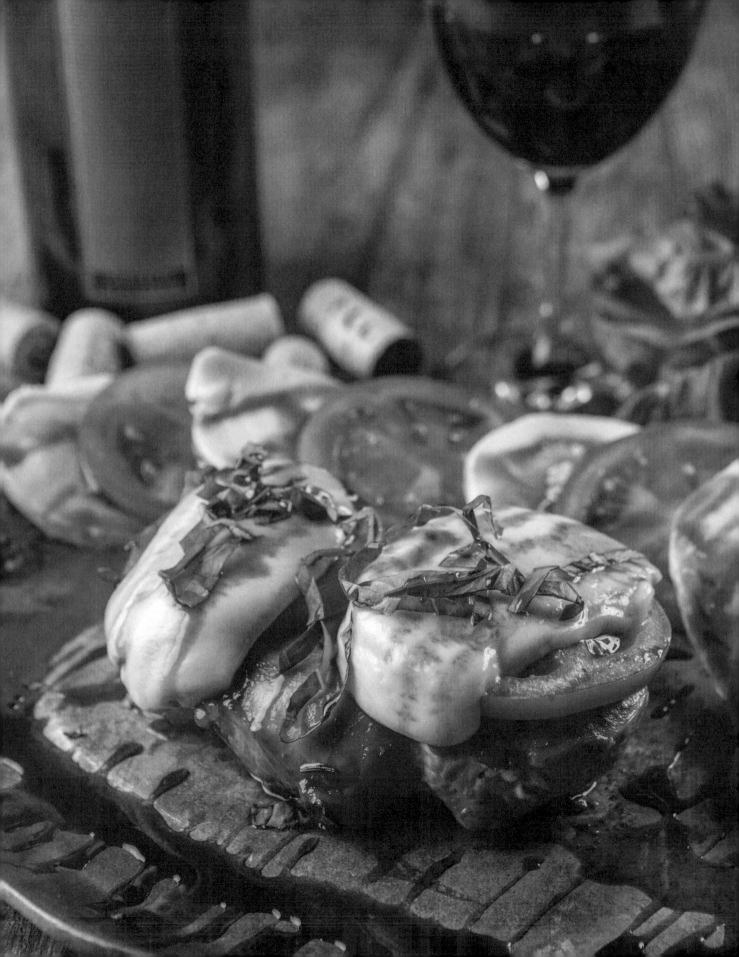

Caprese Grilled Chicken

SERVES 4

We had to include some yard bird—we love chicken! And we love this simple but delicious style of preparing it. With the use of an Oyster Bed Steak Bed, you can get perfectly cooked, juicy chicken every time. If you don't have a Steak Bed yet, we suggest a cast-iron skillet.

¼ cup balsamic vinegar

¼ cup extra virgin olive oil

1 tablespoon Dijon mustard

1 teaspoon honey

1 large garlic clove, grated

¼ teaspoon salt

¼ teaspoon ground black pepper

4 (6-ounce) boneless, skinless chicken breasts

Nonstick cooking spray

1 (8-ounce) fresh mozzarella ball, sliced

1 ripe garden tomato, sliced

¼ cup sliced fresh basil

¼ cup balsamic reduction

In a large bowl, combine the balsamic vinegar, olive oil, mustard, honey, garlic, salt, and pepper and whisk well. Add the chicken breasts and turn to coat. Cover and refrigerate for at least 2 hours—overnight is better.

Preheat your grill (we use a Traeger) to 350°F. Spray an Oyster Bed Steak Bed or cast-iron skillet with nonstick spray. Set the Steak Bed or skillet on the grill. When it is hot, add the chicken and cook until cooked through, 2–4 minutes per side. Top with the fresh mozzarella and tomato and let it heat until the cheese just starts to melt. Transfer to plates and serve topped with the basil and a drizzle of balsamic reduction.

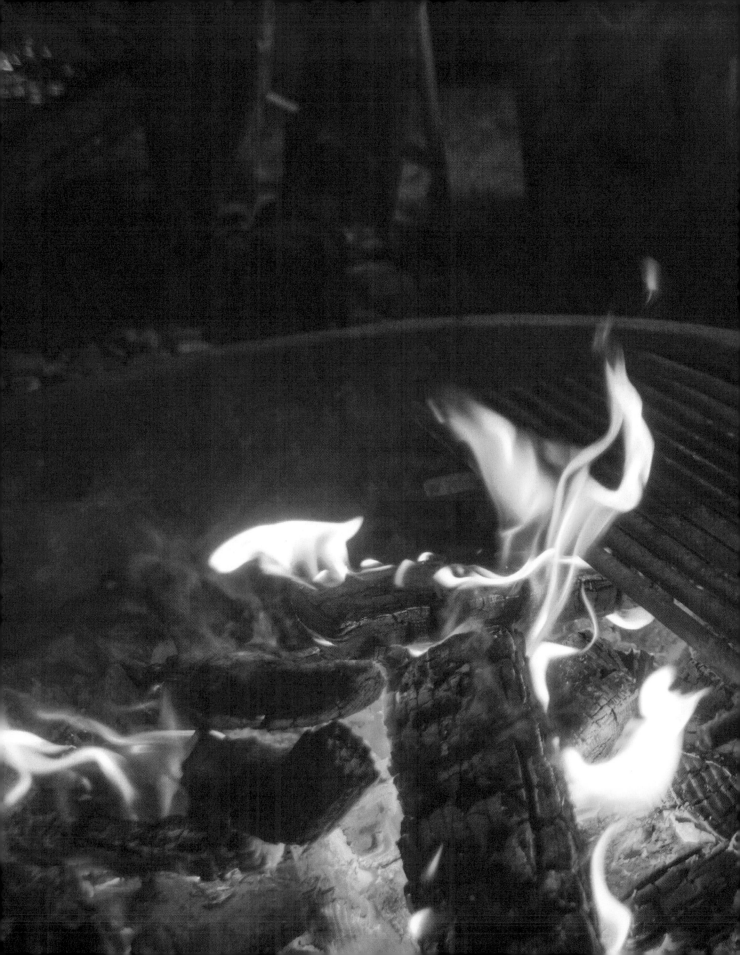

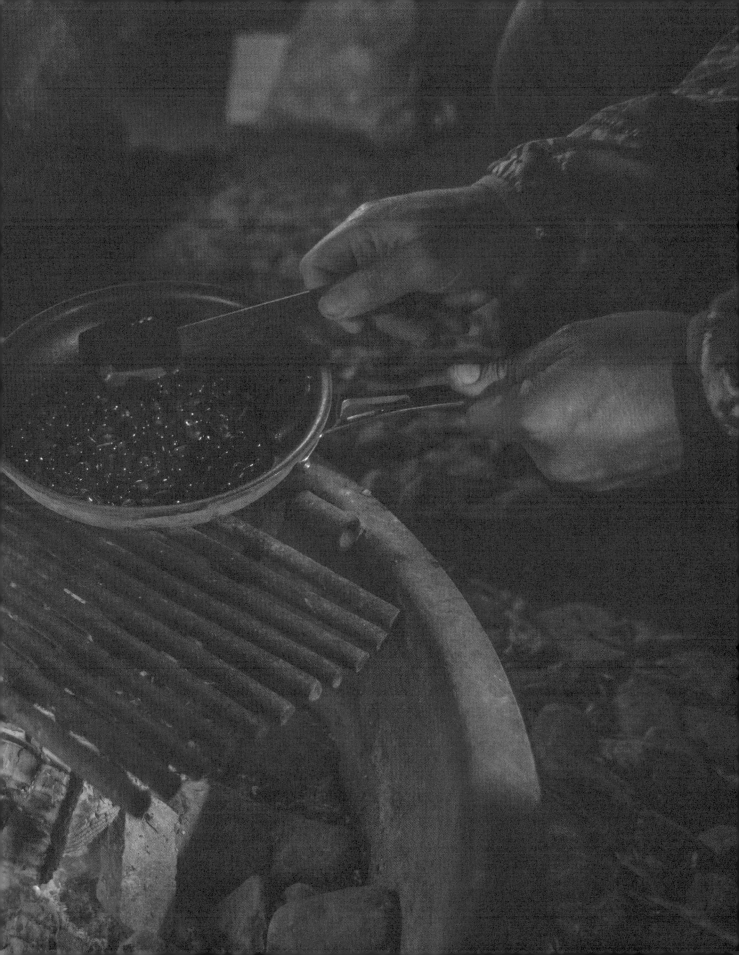

Honey-Soy Marinated Flank Steak

SERVES 6

Brian Grant lived a few houses down from Chad Mendes's family back in Sacramento. We became really close friends with him and his family. We would take turns having cookouts and loved spending time together. Brian got his first Traeger grill around that time, and man did he master that sucker! Here is one of his family's favorite beef recipes, a super easy, East Asian–inspired marinade that works well with just about any kind of red meat. The mix of sweet and savory combined with the smoky flavors of the grill are just amazing. Add these succulent steak strips to salads or tacos or serve alongside your favorite rice dish!

½ cup olive oil

¼ cup soy sauce

¼ cup honey

2 tablespoons red wine vinegar

1 tablespoon garlic salt

1 tablespoon ground ginger

1 (2- to 3-pound) beef flank steak

In a large bowl, combine the olive oil, soy sauce, honey, red wine vinegar, garlic salt, and ginger and whisk well. With a sharp knife, make several shallow slits all over the flank steak and submerge it completely in the marinade. Cover and refrigerate for 8 hours.

When you're ready to cook, preheat your grill (we use a Traeger) to 350°F. Remove the steak from the marinade and place it directly on the grill grate. Grill until the internal temperature hits 140°F (5–10 minutes on each side) for medium rare, or to your desired doneness. Transfer to a cutting board and tent loosely with aluminum foil. Let the steak rest for about 10 minutes, then cut into strips.

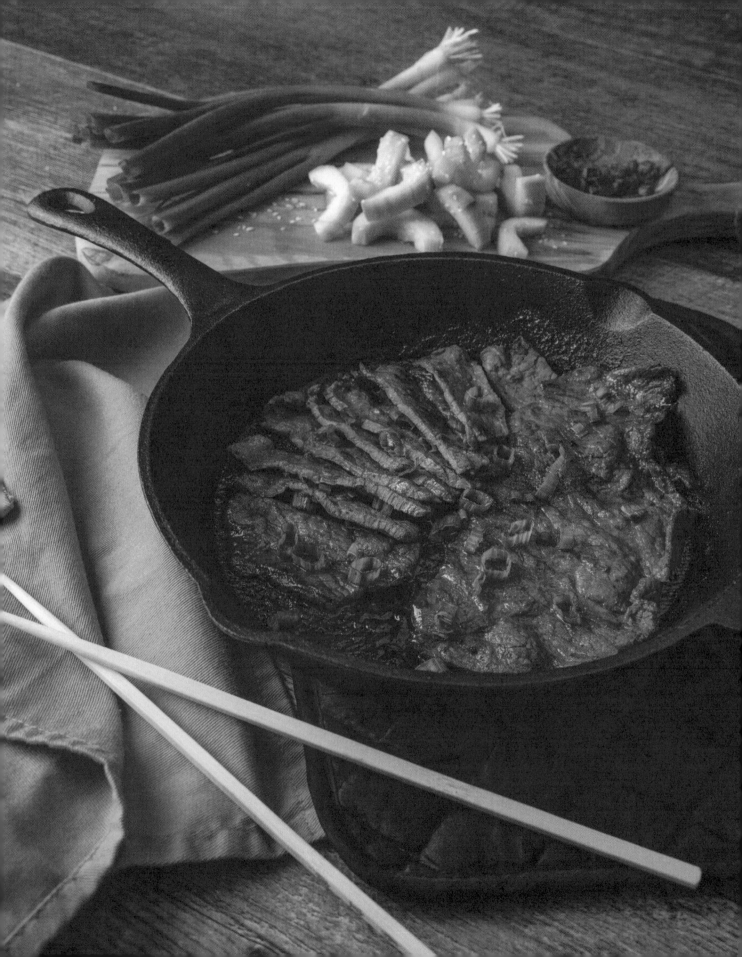

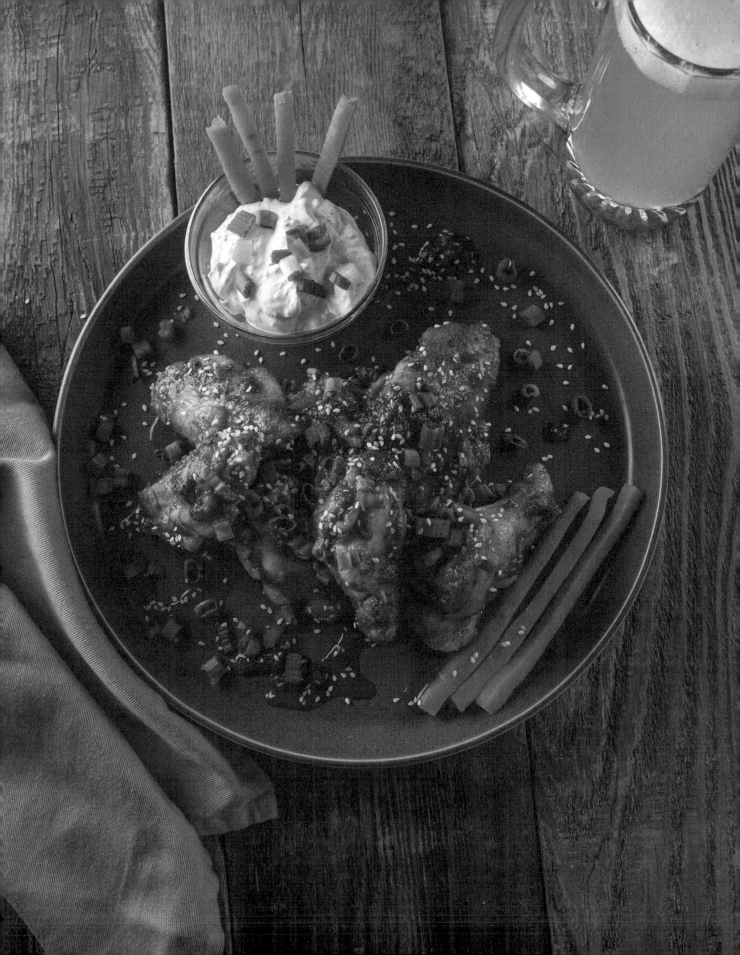

Honey Chipotle Wings

SERVES 4

Everyone loves wings! We all try not to look like first-time eaters when we stuff our faces with them. We love them breaded. We love them with just crispy skin. We love them with sauce. We love them with a dry rub. OK, we love everything about chicken wings! This is one of our all-time favorite recipes. Just be warned: Stock up on napkins.

3 pounds chicken wings, separated into flats and drumettes

1 tablespoon baking powder

1 tablespoon ancho chile powder

1 teaspoon kosher salt

3 canned chipotles in adobo sauce, plus 1 tablespoon adobo sauce

½ cup honey

2 tablespoons fresh lime juice

2 tablespoons soy sauce

1 tablespoon chopped fresh cilantro, for garnish

Set a wire rack over a rimmed baking sheet. Rinse the chicken wings and pat dry with paper towels.

Combine the baking powder, ancho chile powder, and salt in a large bowl. Add the wings and toss to evenly coat them in the rub mixture. Arrange the wings in a single layer on the prepared wire rack. Refrigerate uncovered for 8 hours.

Set up your grill (we use a Traeger) for indirect cooking, with the hot side at 300°F.

While the grill is heating up, combine the chipotles in adobo and adobo sauce, honey, lime juice, and soy sauce in a blender and puree until smooth. Pour the glaze into a large bowl.

Place the wings on the cool side of the grill and cook until they reach an internal temperature of 175°F, about 20–30 minutes, flipping halfway. Transfer the wings to the bowl of glaze and toss until they are evenly coated. Return the wings to the grill over direct heat and increase the heat to 450°F. Once the wings start to slightly char, transfer them to a platter, sprinkle with the chopped cilantro, and serve.

Archery Elk Hunt

Chad Mendes

After I harvested my first backcountry bull, Oregon quickly became one of my favorite places to chase elk. In 2018 I was lucky enough to harvest my first Oregon bull with a bow. Our Finz and Featherz crew teamed up with Casey from Opal Butte Outfitters that year and brought in a handful of clients to chase screaming bulls. I wasn't going to pass up this opportunity and quickly jumped in to hunt with everyone. Abby, this time a few weeks pregnant with our daughter Lula, decided at the last minute she wanted to join us on the adventure, so we headed up to northern Oregon once again.

After four days of chasing screaming bulls and so many close calls, my arrow finally connected on a giant. The afternoon started off with me and Abby climbing up in a double setup tree stand. We were positioned about 30 yards above a heavily used wallow. After about an hour of sitting, a cow elk came in to drink and we caught a glimpse or two of a mature bull in the timber with no shot. I had a great feeling about this spot. As the wind started to pick up right around prime time, I looked back at Abby and noticed her knuckles were white and her

face was pale. The movement of the tree and the height of the tree stand had her terrified. She finally looked at me and said, "I can't do it anymore. I'm gonna get down and hike up to service and see if someone can come grab me." It was prime time to sit, but I did what any loving husband would do . . . no, I didn't. I was a jerk and let her go alone!

After about ten more minutes of sitting and fearing the worst—worrying that she might run into a mountain lion or bear—I got down and started hiking, thinking I'd meet back up with her. By the time I got to the top of the mountain, she was already gone. My phone rang, and on the other end of the line was my buddy Dave, saying, "You need to haul ass down here! We have Abby and we are in the middle of a bull frenzy!"

It was about an hour before dark when Dave and I started sneaking in. We could hear bulls bugling about 200 yards away. We crept closer and closer until we looked up and saw Abby and our two buddies sitting about 50 yards above us on the hillside in the timber. Dave let out a cow call to get their attention. All three looked down at us and pointed toward the meadow on the other side of the hill, mouthing the word "Elk!"

Little did we know, that single cow call that Dave let out caught the attention of a stud bull. I could hear multiple herds of elk in the meadow just 100 yards away. I took my boots off and nocked an arrow. I slowly started to climb toward all the commotion. As my eyes began to crest the hill, I immediately caught sight of ivory tips from a bull's antlers—just like my backcountry hunt a few years before. This time, though, I could tell he was looking back behind him toward the rest of the elk. I slowly ranged the tree next to him at 43 yards and set my pin. In complete ninja mode, I climbed the hill just a tad more so when I stood up I would be able to see all his vitals clearly. I knew he wasn't going to stay put long, but I also knew that if I rushed and made too much noise he was gone. After about 5 yards of climbing hunched over, I came to full draw and slowly sat up. Right as my pin settled behind his shoulder he turned and looked right at me but it was too late. My arrow found its home and down he went. I had just harvested one of my biggest bulls to date with my wife, unborn daughter, and some close buddies right there with me. It's a hunt I'll never forget!

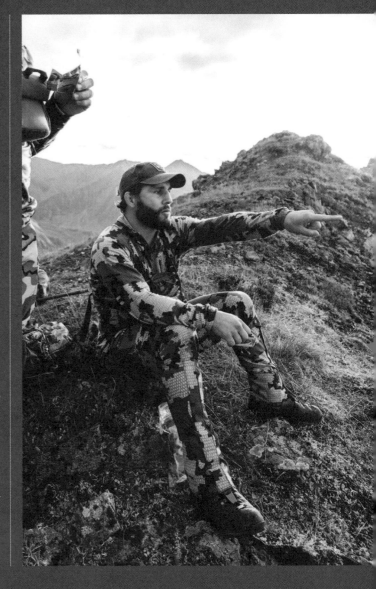

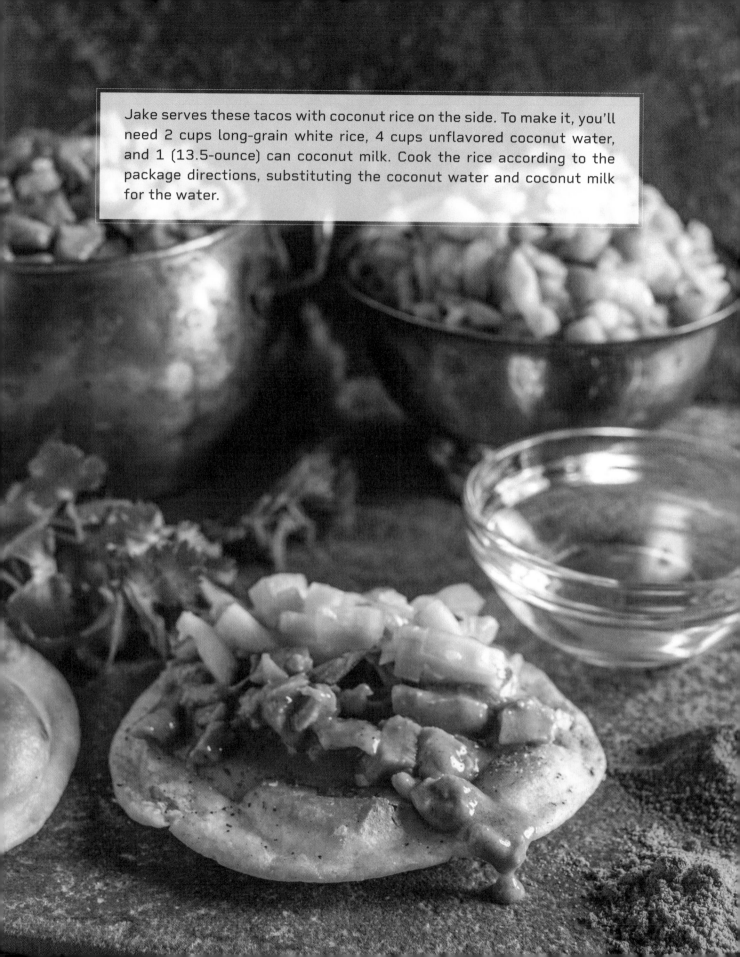

Jake serves these tacos with coconut rice on the side. To make it, you'll need 2 cups long-grain white rice, 4 cups unflavored coconut water, and 1 (13.5-ounce) can coconut milk. Cook the rice according to the package directions, substituting the coconut water and coconut milk for the water.

Chicken Curry Tacos

MAKES 10 TACOS

Chad Mendes met his friend Jake Hodges on an airplane a few years ago. We were both flying to Utah to shoot in the Total Archery Challenge and found out we lived only a couple miles apart! Jake is a firefighter who loves the outdoors and loves to cook. Chad fondly remembers the night he and Abby joined Jake and his wife for dinner, and his friend made these amazing curry tacos. Chad's mouth waters every time he thinks about that meal! Jake was kind enough to share the recipe.

CUCUMBER SLAW

3 large cucumbers, peeled and diced

1 red onion, diced

½ bunch cilantro, chopped

2 teaspoons sugar

¼ teaspoon ground ginger

Salt to taste

Pinch cayenne pepper (optional)

¼ cup white wine vinegar

TACOS

4 pounds boneless, skinless chicken thighs, trimmed of excess fat

5 tablespoons curry powder, divided

Salt and ground black pepper to taste

1 teaspoon ground ginger

1 (13.5-ounce) can coconut milk

10 small flour tortillas

Sriracha sauce

In a large bowl, combine the cucumber, red onion, and cilantro. Sprinkle with the sugar, ginger, salt, and cayenne pepper if you want some heat. Drizzle with the white wine vinegar and stir well. Cover and refrigerate for up to a few hours until ready to serve.

Preheat your grill (we use a Traeger) to 450°F.

Sprinkle the chicken thighs all over with 2 tablespoons of the curry powder and season with salt and pepper. Grill the chicken, turning once or twice, until cooked through, 2–4 minutes per side. Transfer the thighs to a cutting board and cut into ½-inch pieces.

Put the chicken in a large saucepan and add the remaining 3 tablespoons curry powder, ginger, and coconut milk. Simmer over medium-high heat for 10 minutes.

Meanwhile, in a small frying pan, heat the tortillas over medium heat for 45 seconds on each side.

Serve the chicken mixture on the warm tortillas, topped with cucumber slaw and Sriracha.

Chicken and Smoked Sausage Jambalaya

SERVES 6–8

Chad Mendes's good friend and business partner Mike Pappa and his wife, Olivia, have been a huge part of his life. Creating Finz and Featherz together with Mike brought our families together. We travel the world hunting, fishing, and exploring many different styles of food. Here is a recipe that Olivia makes that will warm your soul on any cold and rainy day!

1½ pounds boneless, skinless chicken breasts and/or thighs, cut into 1-inch pieces

1 teaspoon salt

⅛ teaspoon ground black pepper

⅛ teaspoon cayenne pepper

3 tablespoons vegetable oil

8 ounces Andouille sausage, cut into ½-inch pieces

2 cups chopped yellow onion

1 cup chopped green bell pepper

1 cup chopped celery

4 garlic cloves, minced

3 cups chicken stock

1 (16-ounce) can diced tomatoes, drained with juice reserved

½ cup chopped green onions (green parts only)

2 tablespoons chopped fresh parsley

2 pounds medium shrimp, peeled and deveined

1 teaspoon hot sauce

2 cups long-grain white rice, rinsed and drained

Sprinkle the chicken with the salt, black pepper, and cayenne. Heat the vegetable oil in large, heavy pot or Dutch oven over medium heat. Add the chicken and cook, stirring, until browned, 8–10 minutes. Transfer the chicken to a bowl.

Add the sausage to the pot and cook, stirring, until lightly browned, about 5 minutes. Add the sausage to the chicken in the bowl. Add the onion, bell pepper, celery, and garlic to the pot and cook, scraping the bottom of the pot to loosen any browned bits, until softened, about 5 minutes. Return the chicken and sausage to the pot, reduce the heat to low, cover, and cook for 25 minutes, stirring occasionally.

Add the chicken stock and tomato juice from the can, cover, and simmer for about 45 minutes.

Add the tomatoes, green onions, parsley, shrimp, and hot sauce and adjust the seasonings to taste. Stir in the rice, cover the pot, and bring to a boil. Reduce the heat to medium-low and simmer, stirring occasionally, until the rice is tender and fluffy and all the liquid is absorbed, about 25 minutes. Serve warm.

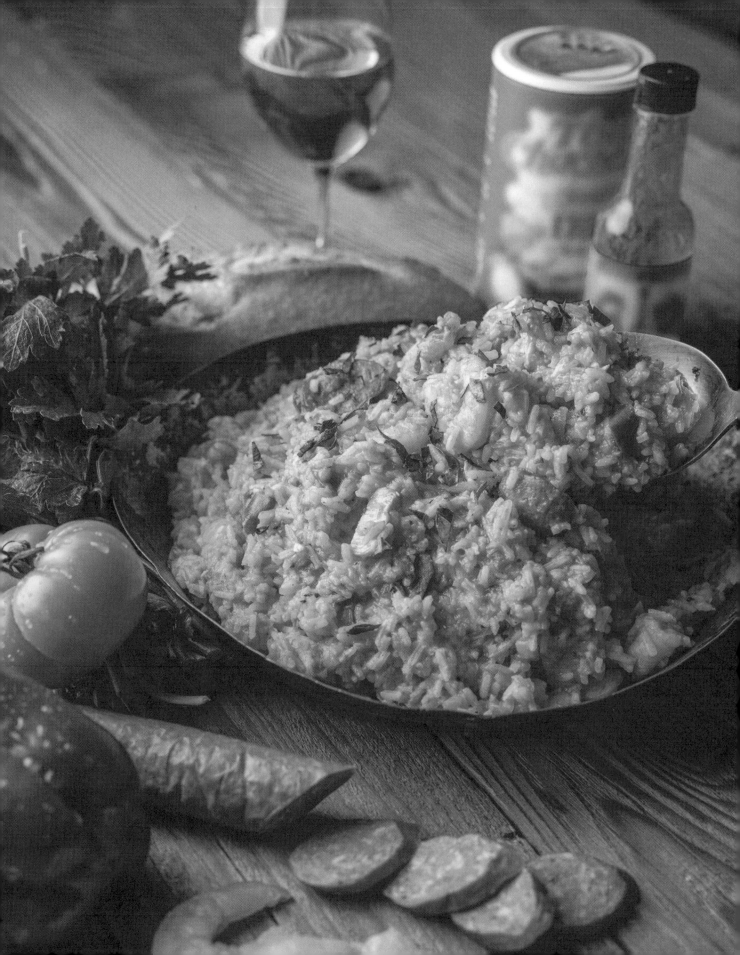

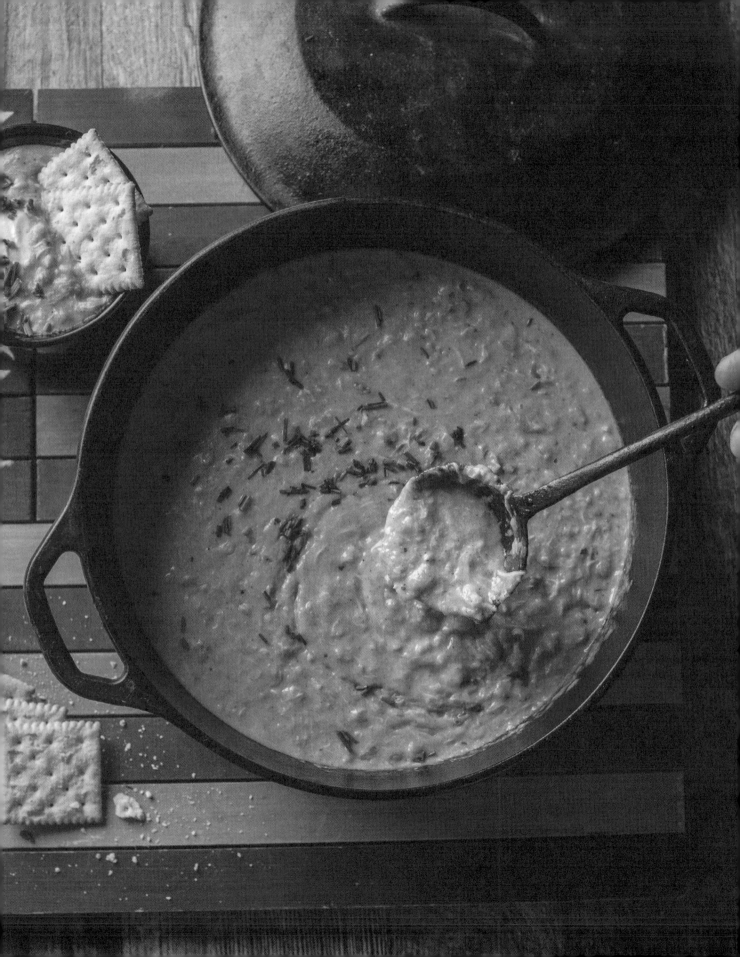

Dan Henderson's White Chicken Chili

SERVES 8-10

Dan Henderson has been a force in the MMA ring and octagon for years, knocking out some of the biggest legends in the sport. His wife has a few KO's under her belt as well, and this hearty white bean and chicken chili is one of them! This recipe is perfect for those rainy, stormy days or in camp after a long hunt. She does recommend bringing your "stretchy pants" for this chili!

8 tablespoons (1 stick) unsalted butter

1 medium white onion, diced

1 heaping tablespoon minced garlic

1 whole rotisserie chicken, skin and bones discarded, meat shredded

1 (15-ounce) can great Northern beans, rinsed and drained

2 (15-ounce) cans creamed corn

1 (4-ounce) can diced green chiles, drained

1 tablespoon chili powder

1 tablespoon cumin

Pinch ground mace

Pinch paprika

Pinch oregano

Salt and ground black pepper to taste

2 (14.5-ounce) cans chicken stock

1 cup half-and-half

¼ cup milk

8 ounces cream cheese

TOPPINGS

Sour cream

Shredded pepper Jack cheese

Sliced green onions

Melt the butter in a large pot over medium heat. Add the onion and cook for about 5 minutes, until soft. Stir in the garlic and cook for 2 minutes, or until fragrant. Add the chicken, beans, corn, chiles, seasonings, and chicken stock. Stir well and simmer for 2 hours (while you put on your stretch pants). Toward the end of cooking, stir in the half-and-half, milk, and cream cheese and let cook just until hot.

Serve in bowls. Load on some sour cream, shredded cheese, and green onions.

Hendo says: "Don't forget corn bread muffins for the side."

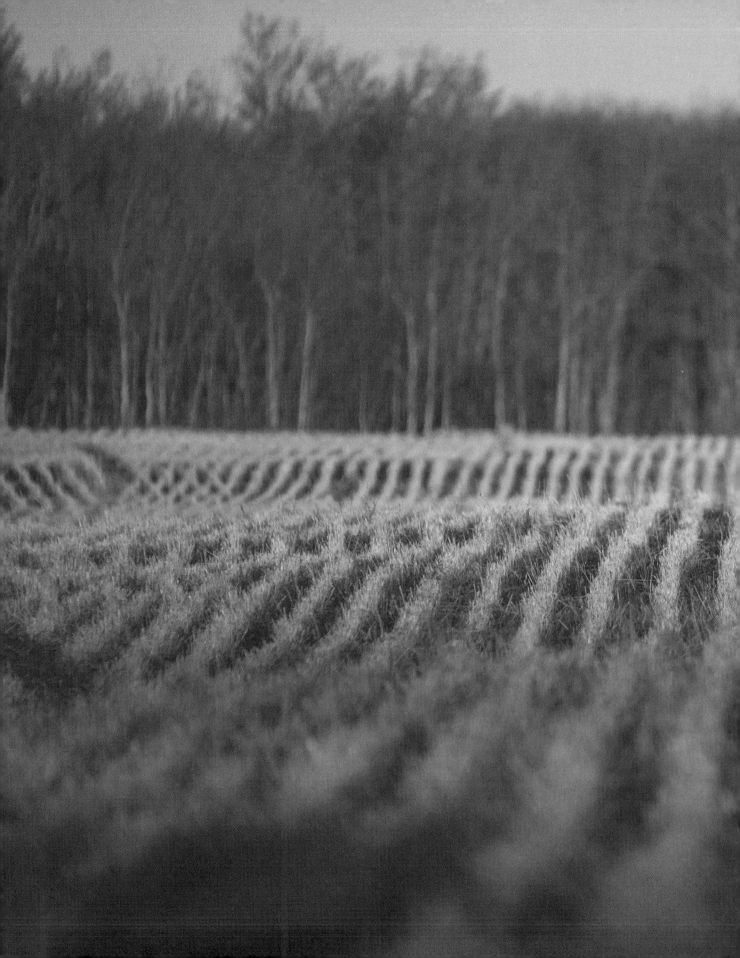

SIDES AND SAUCES

As a kid growing up in northern Nevada, Clay Belding, Chad's brother, knew that the smells of summer that filled the air in the backyard were of fresh flowers, grass, onions, garlic, and manure. Clay can remember helping his dad shovel new soil that was dumped on the driveway and wheeling it back to the garden. (Clay mostly dug tunnels in the new dirt and made double the work for his dad as he got to ride the empty wheelbarrow back to the driveway.) Finding worms in the fresh soil was like finding gold. He wanted to see how many he could find, and the bigger the better. Looking back now, that garden wasn't big, but it always provided fresh food, enough for our family and fond memories of a simple life.

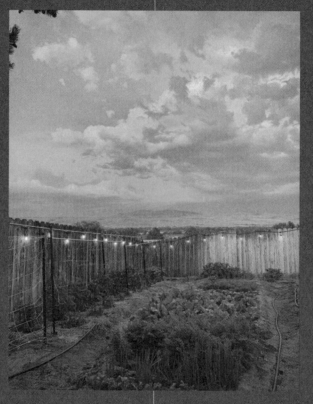

As the years passed by and family life got busy with school, careers, and kids, the garden turned into a basketball court so the Belding brothers could show each other who was the best athlete of the family. Fast-forward twenty years, the Belding parents retired and moved to their dream spot, and Clay built a log cabin for them to spend their golden years in. The first thing his dad did was put in a new garden! Memories of years past rushed back, reminding us all what this new garden would provide for our family.

August 1, 2006, was opening day of archery antelope season in Nevada, and my dad drew a coveted tag! My brother Clint and I tagged along for the first week of the hunt in hopes of seeing our dad tag-out on a trophy Nevada speed goat. As the first week passed, and with no luck in sight for our dad, Clint and I had to head home for prior obligations, while Dad wanted to stay one more day to try to fill his tag. As we pulled out of camp, Dad said, "Please take care of the garden when you get home. I love you!" The next afternoon, August 9, 2006, with a hoe in hand working my dad's garden, I heard my phone ring. It was not the call I expected or wanted. I learned of my father's passing and my life forever changed.

Ten years later I was fortunate enough to purchase my first home and, yes, the first thing I did was build a garden. I forgot how much I loved the smell of the onions, garlic, and tomatoes that filled the summer air when I was a child. We all sat down as a family and talked about what seeds we wanted to plant. I even turned the worms that we purchased into a science lesson for the kids before we placed them into the soil. It was all starting to happen; the memories of my childhood were coming to life for our children. I could only hope that the excitement and happiness I had in my dad's garden would be felt with my kids. Let me tell you, it was! Every passing year, our garden is the talk of the family! We all get giddy when "Garden Time" rolls around each year.

In northern Nevada, we get all four seasons, so when it comes to gardening, we have to be very careful when to plant. Too soon and the frost can kill your plants; too late means not enough time in the dirt and no bounty. As with much in life, timing is everything. When you hit it perfectly, you just sit back and smile!

As spring gives way to summer and the temperatures rise, growth starts to happen fast! We go from watering once a day to twice a day to almost three. The brown soil is now covered in green. All that hard work and waiting we did in the spring is starting to pay off. But that was just the beginning of hard work. Now we need to build a trellis for the tomatoes and cucumbers, and fix the soil from water runoff, and pull weeds, and fertilize, and pick the bounty, and, and, and. . . . All while being outside with our family away from the phones, computers, and TVs. It was happening—the sights and smells of my childhood, which I missed so much, were all coming back as I watched the smiles on my kids' faces.

Before we knew it, our tomatoes grew over our heads, the deep color of the beets was peeking through the dirt, the peppers almost breaking their stems, the corn, okra, onions, lettuce, radishes, potatoes, squash, and carrots were all feeding our family and friends. We had more vegetables than we could even imagine. We are Providers. All I can say is, "Thank you, Dad. I am taking care of the garden. I love you too!"

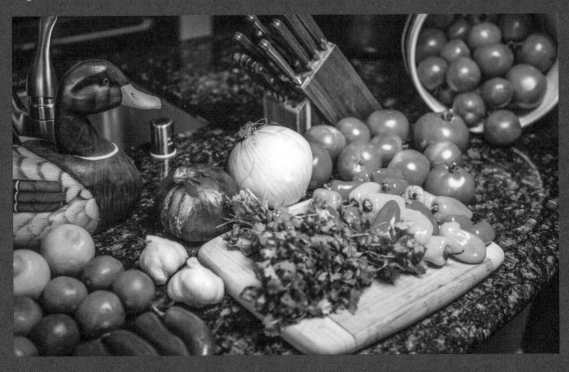

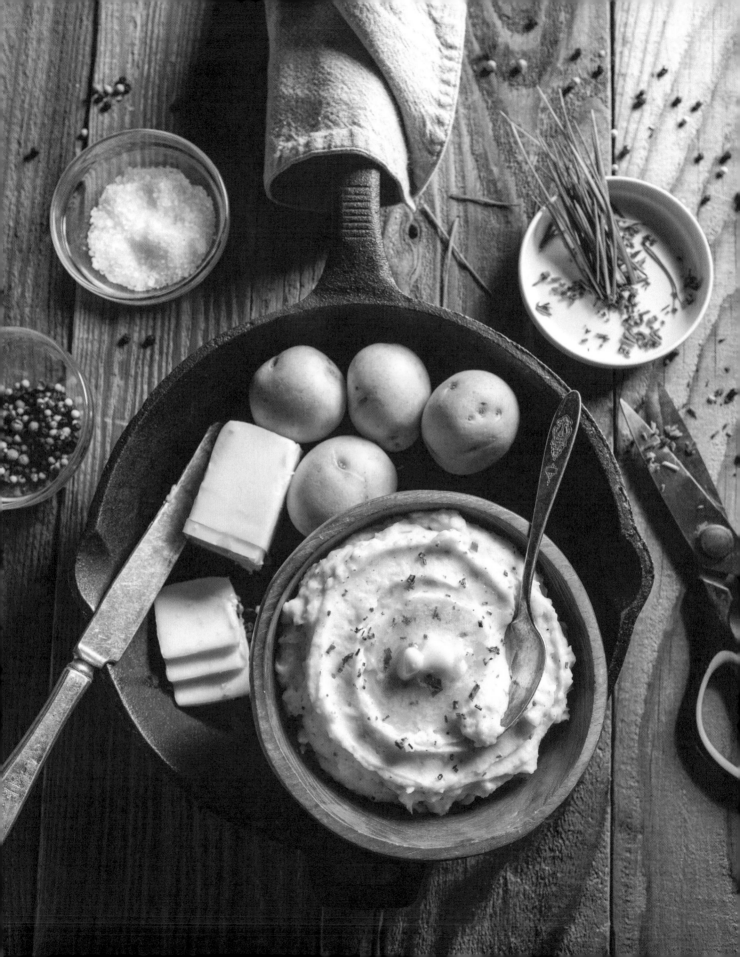

Ranch Mashers

SERVES 4

Wondering what to make to go with all that ground meat in your freezer? Here it is! Mix these creamy ranch potatoes with your favorite veggies and ground meat for a meal that will stick to your ribs and blow your mind with flavor!

---

3 pounds small yellow potatoes, halved

4 tablespoons (½ stick) unsalted butter

¾ cup sour cream

1 (1-ounce) packet ranch salad dressing and seasoning mix

1½ teaspoons ground black pepper

1½ teaspoons garlic powder

Salt to taste

2 tablespoons minced fresh chives

Put the potatoes in a large pot and pour in enough water to cover them by about an inch. Bring to a boil and cook until the potatoes slide off a fork when poked, about 10 minutes. Drain. Add the butter, sour cream, ranch seasoning, pepper, and garlic powder. Mash and stir the mixture. Taste and add salt to your liking. Transfer to a serving bowl and garnish with the chives. Enjoy!

Chad Mendes says: "You can adjust the thickness of your mashed potatoes by using more or less sour cream."

Dianna's Macaroni Salad

SERVES 8-10

The name Belding is known in hunting. The name Belding has been known in baseball. But the main area of this world that the name Belding has become famous for is Aunt Dianna's Macaroni Salad! Everybody has eaten this type of dish, but this is the only version we have ever tasted that makes us want to constantly see it in front of us. We beg Aunt Dianna to bring it to every BBQ and family gathering. You would think with the size of the bowl she carries it in, there would be leftovers . . . never the case!

Garlic salt

1 pound elbow macaroni

1 cup mayonnaise

¼ cup pickle juice

1 teaspoon yellow mustard

6–8 sweet pickles, chopped

8–10 dill pickles, chopped

1 red onion, diced

4 hard-boiled eggs, sliced

Ground black pepper

Bring a large pot of water to a boil and stir in a good amount of garlic salt. Cook the macaroni according to the package directions. Drain and rinse under cold running water. Drain well.

In a large bowl, mix the mayo, pickle juice, and mustard. Add the pickles and onion. Stir in the macaroni. Place the hard-boiled eggs on top. Sprinkle with pepper.

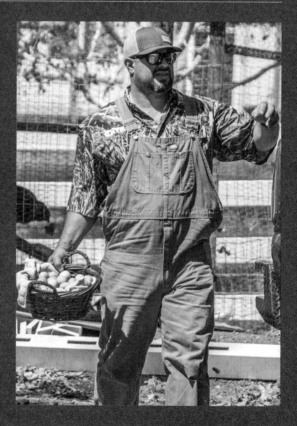

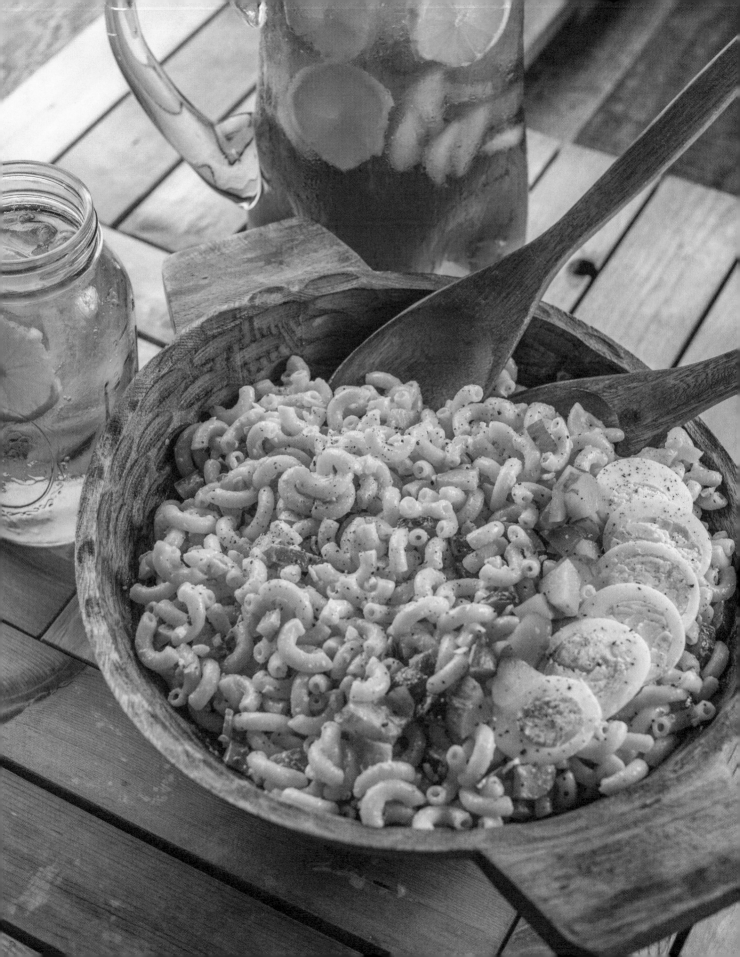

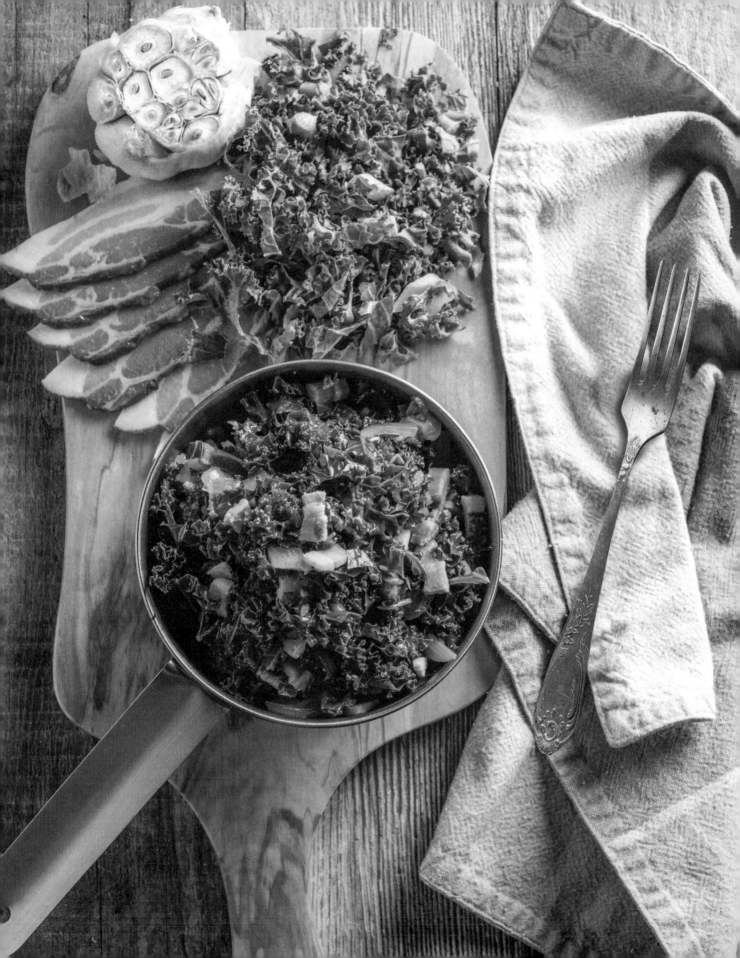

Cobb's Collards

SERVES 6-8

We love tradition. And we love the South! This is a Cobb family staple from the great state of Georgia. These collard greens hit the spot when they accompany our favorite chicken fry or even when they stand alone. And in the words of the magical Brent Cobb, "Just don't forget to serve the pot liquor (broth) with corn bread. And none of that sugar bread. The real stuff!" Yep, what he said!

---

3 tablespoons olive oil

½ medium onion, diced

1 tablespoon minced garlic

1 smoked ham hock

5 cups chicken stock

2 cups water

1 teaspoon crushed red pepper

1 (2-pound) bag prewashed chopped collard greens

Heat the olive oil in a large pot over medium-low heat. Add the onion and garlic and cook, stirring occasionally, until tender, about 10 minutes. Add the ham hock, chicken stock, water, and crushed red pepper. Increase the heat to bring the mixture to a boil. Cover, reduce the heat, and simmer for 20 minutes.

Stir in the collards, a handful at a time. Cover and simmer for 2 hours.

Fish out the ham hock and debone. Chop up the meat and stir it back into the greens. Enjoy!

Caesar Salad

SERVES 4–6

This recipe comes to us courtesy of Jim Rhea, whose stepfather, Ed Rodden, taught him the recipe. Ed was a gentleman rancher from Oakdale, California. He often had buddies over prior to dinner for a scotch or gin depending on the time of the year. They traded stories and cooking tips. Ed told the story of a man named Caesar Cardini, an Italian immigrant who opened a restaurant in Tijuana, Mexico, to avoid the rules of Prohibition. Apparently, some Hollywood stars of the time, also looking to escape the laws of Prohibition, traveled south of the border and would frequent his place. On one occasion his establishment was busier than normal, and Caesar was forced to improvise. He made a salad dressing with what he had on hand . . . and the rest is history.

Jim says, "I have eaten hundreds of Caesar salads from many restaurants, and this recipe has been my favorite, and what I believe to be fairly close to the original. The measurements below are estimates at best. Adjust to your taste. I never saw Ed measure ingredients for this, always by feel. But it was mandatory that it was served on chilled plates or bowls!"

---

6 tablespoons extra virgin olive oil

2 tablespoons red wine vinegar

2 large egg yolks (see note)

1 tablespoon Dijon mustard

Dash Worcestershire sauce

Dash hot sauce

Juice of 1 lime

2 garlic cloves, pressed

3–4 anchovy fillets, chopped and mashed into a paste

3 romaine lettuce hearts

Shaved or freshly grated parmesan cheese

Croutons

In a large stainless-steel bowl, combine the olive oil, red wine vinegar, egg yolks, Dijon, Worcestershire, hot sauce, and lime juice. Whisk well until emulsified. Whisk in the garlic. Add the mashed anchovies. Cover and refrigerate the dressing to chill for a bit.

When ready, separate the romaine leaves. (Use whole leaves or tear them, don't chop.) Toss the romaine with the dressing, then add the parmesan. Top with croutons.

Jim says: "Put 2 whole eggs in boiling water for a minute and a half, then separate out the yolks."

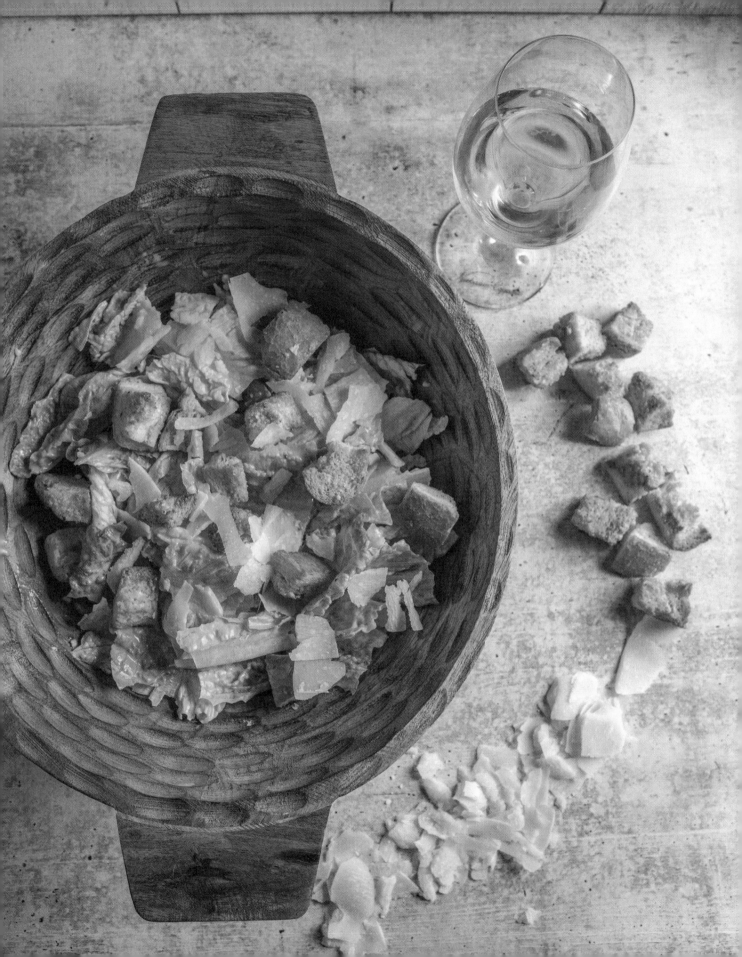

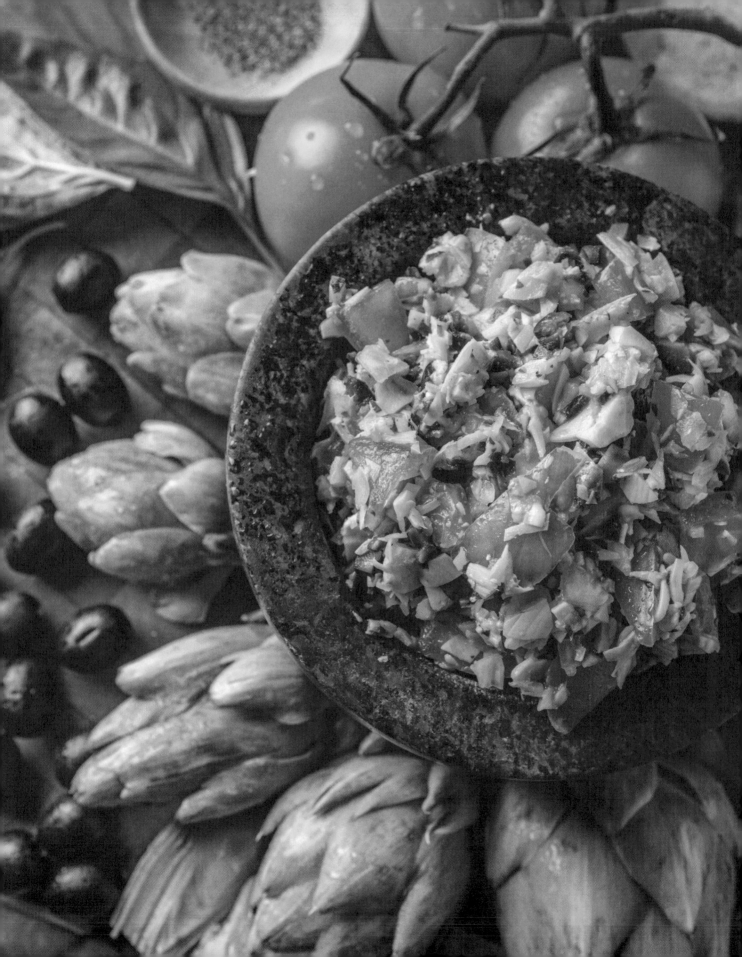

Chunky Artichoke Salsa

SERVES 6-8

Chad Belding's brother Clay is a Provider. He can hunt. He can prepare meat. Heck, he can even butcher an entire elk! On top of all of that, he might be best known for his garden. That is where this salsa recipe originated, and he has it mastered. Trust us, you can make as much as your garden will produce, but it will all be gone before most of your guests arrive!

---

1 (6.5-ounce) jar chopped marinated
    artichoke hearts, undrained

¼ cup pitted ripe olives, chopped

2 tablespoons chopped red onion

3 medium plum tomatoes, diced

1 garlic clove, pressed

2 tablespoons snipped fresh basil leaves

Salt and ground pepper to taste

Tortilla chips, for serving

Drain the marinade from the artichokes into a mixing bowl. Add the artichoke hearts, olives, onion, tomatoes, garlic, and basil and mix gently. Season with salt and pepper. Serve with your favorite chips.

Artichoke Bruschetta

Preheat the oven to 400°F. Thinly slice a French baguette. Spoon the salsa onto the slices and top with grated parmesan cheese. Place the bruschetta on a rimmed baking sheet and bake until the bread is crispy, about 10 minutes.

Loftin's Mississippi Tomato Gravy

SERVES 4

If you've got 'em, a quart of homegrown canned tomatoes makes this sauce extra special. This recipe comes to us courtesy of Leith Loftin. We like to serve it over our favorite biscuits with eggs.

¼ cup bacon grease or vegetable oil

2 heaping tablespoons all-purpose flour

1 (28-ounce) can diced tomatoes

Salt and ground black pepper to taste

In a large pot, heat the bacon grease over low heat. Whisk in the flour and cook, stirring, until it becomes a thick paste. Add the tomatoes with their juice and increase the heat to medium; bring to a boil. Reduce the heat and simmer till ready to eat. Season with salt and pepper.

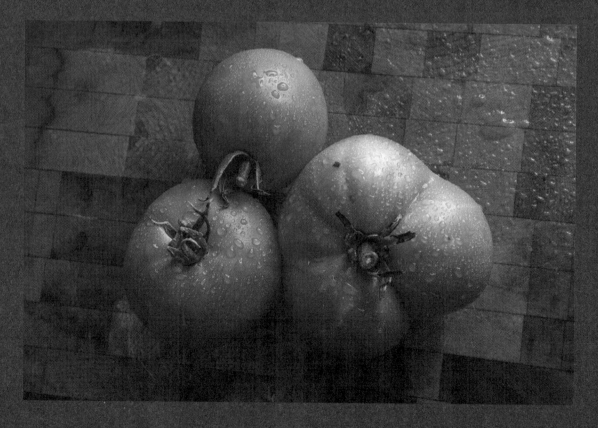

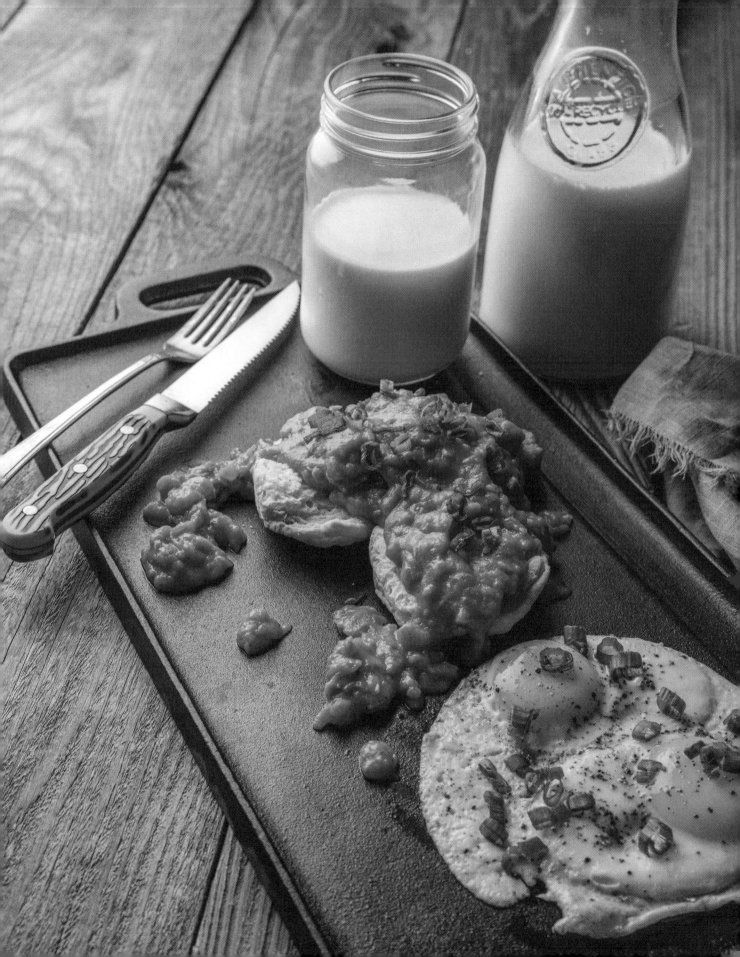

Cocktails

The Macon

2 canned peach slices
1 tablespoon vanilla simple syrup
½ cup unsweetened iced tea

1 ounce Jack Daniel's Old No. 7 Tennessee Whiskey
Splash club soda

Muddle the peaches and simple syrup in the bottom of a rocks glass. Add ice. Pour the tea and whiskey over the rocks. Gently stir to combine the ingredients and top with a splash of club soda.

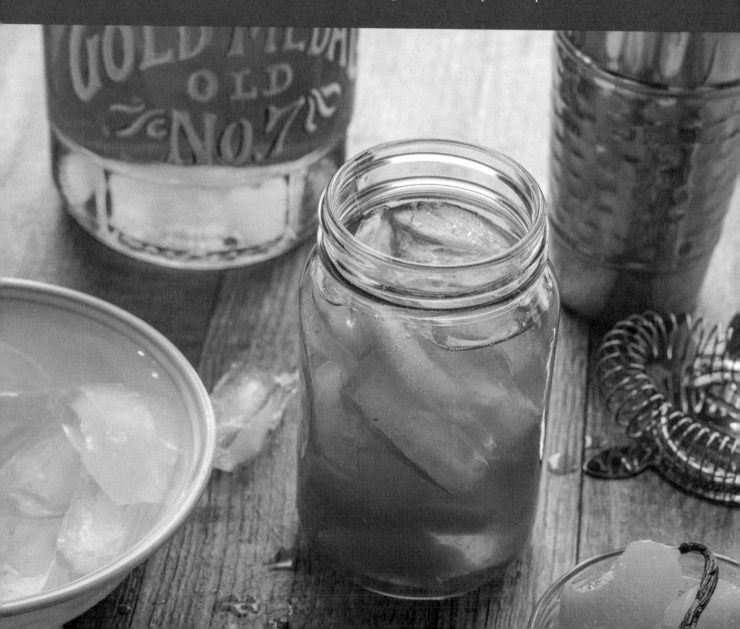

Country Club

1 ounce Gentleman Jack
Splash cherry juice
Splash bitters
Splash club soda
1 maraschino cherry

Fill a glass to the rim with ice. Add the whiskey, cherry juice, and bitters. Top with club soda and gently stir. Garnish with a cherry.

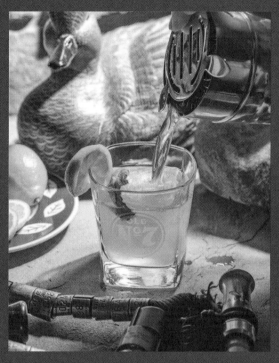

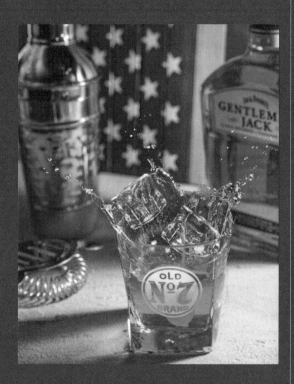

The Honey Hole

10 fresh mint leaves
½ lemon, cut into wedges
1 ounce Jack Daniel's Tennessee Honey
½ cup lemonade
Splash club soda

Muddle the mint leaves and lemon at the bottom of a rocks glass. Add ice. Pour the whiskey and lemonade over the rocks. Swirl to incorporate all the ingredients together, then top with a splash of club soda.

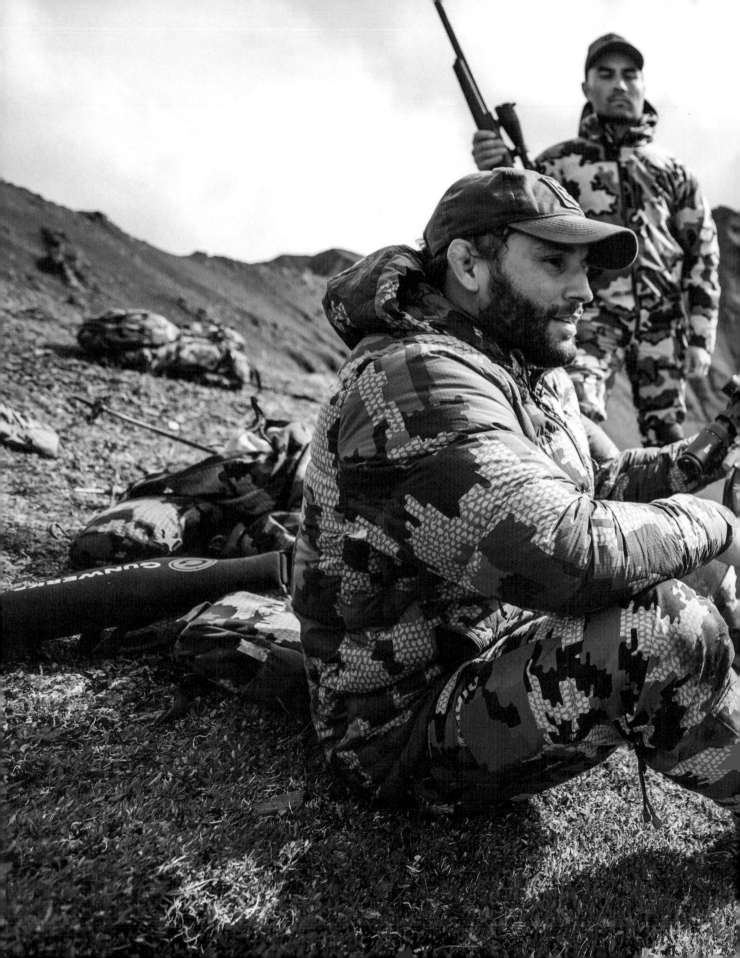

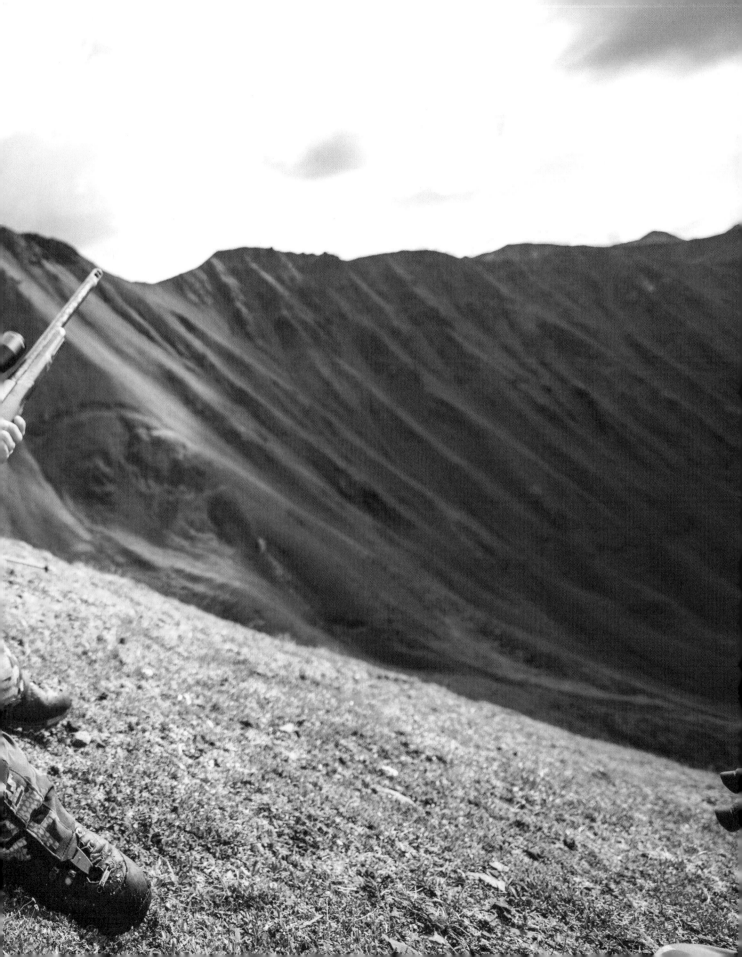

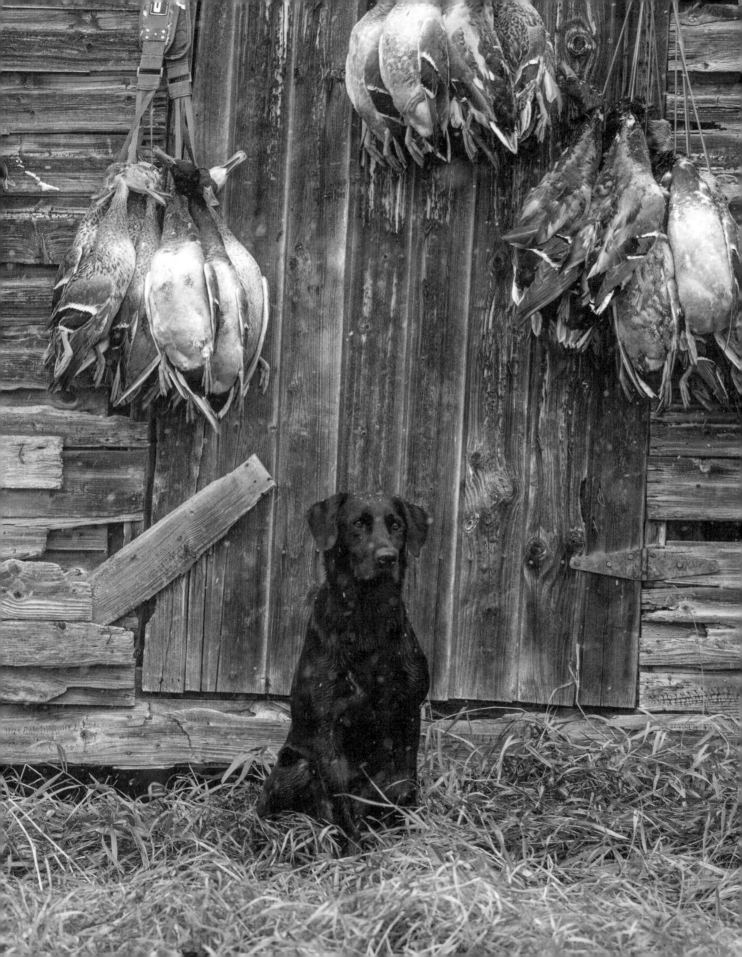

ACKNOWLEDGMENTS

We'd like to thank everyone who made this book a reality.

The team at 3 Arts: Richard Abate, Mark Schulman, and Martha Stevens

At BenBella Books: Glenn Yeffeth, Leah Wilson, Claire Schulz, Sarah Avinger, Jessika Rieck, and Jennifer Canzoneri

All those who generously contributed recipes: Brad and Ellen Arington, Paul Basso, Dianna Belding, Billy Bogey, Rihana Cary, Brent Cobb, Kristy Crabtree, Alex Crosby, Chelly Cross, Glenn Fillipone, Brad Forsythe, Brian Grant, JT Harden, Jake Hodges, Brian Laird, Leith Loftin, Olivia Pappa, Mike Parker, Judy Raines, Jim Rhea, and Jennifer Swenson

On our team: Clay Belding, Tom Rassuchine, and Jennifer Swenson

Andy Perwin and Christy Crabtree for graciously donating their home for the photo shoot

And most importantly, our families and good friends: Orville and Faith Belding; Clint and Heather Belding; Alyssa Ryley Belding; Chase Belding; Chance Belding; Clay Belding; Caden Belding; Chance and Ashleigh Henderson; Emma Braunstein; Mel and Dianna Belding; Les Naisbitt; Mike and Kristie Marchese; Jim and Julie Rhea; Glenn, Clarita, Vinnie, and Bella Fillipone; Abby Mendes; Lula Mendes; Nicole, Ewan, and Fiona Burger; and Judy Raines. You make us proud to be Providers.

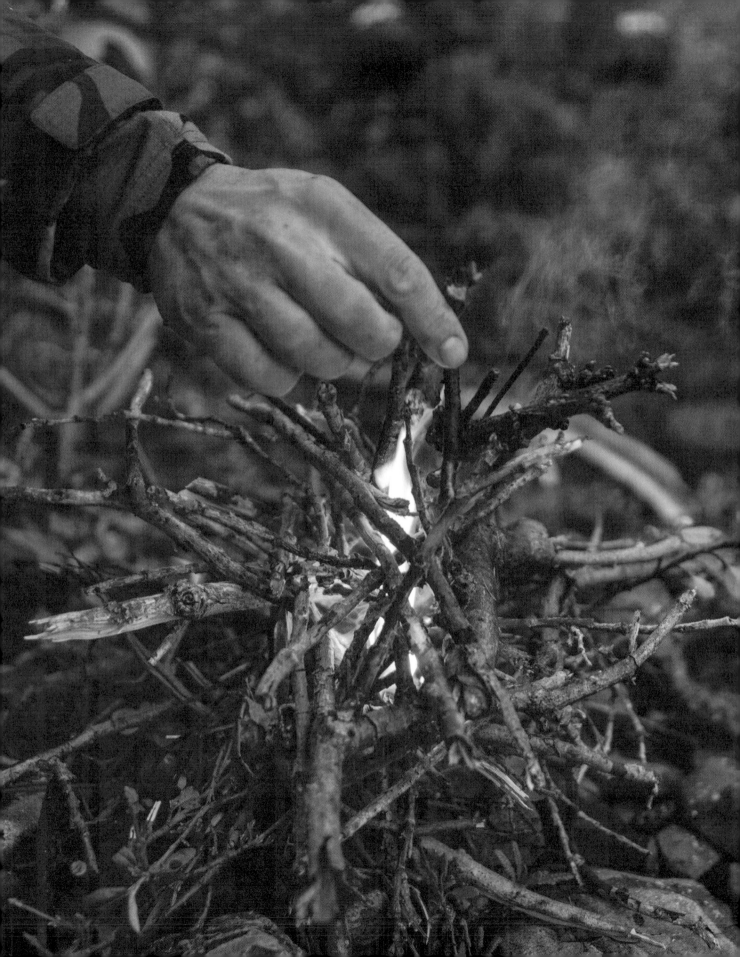

INDEX

RECIPE AND KEY INGREDIENT INDEX

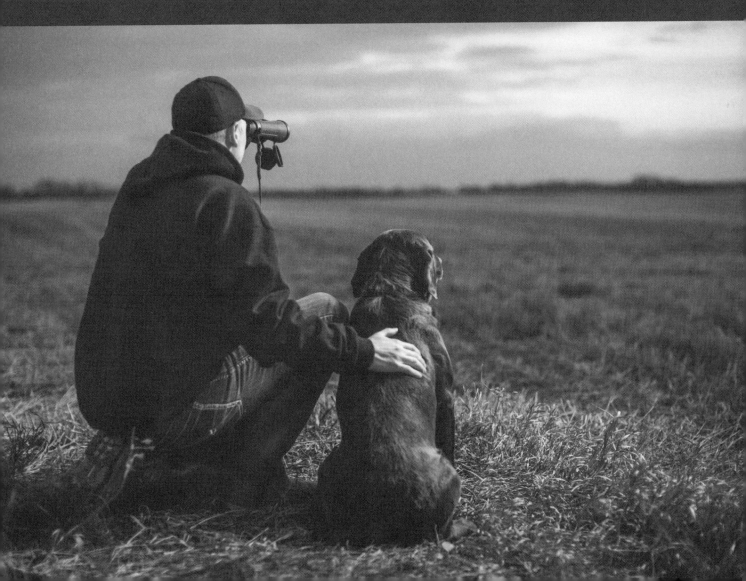

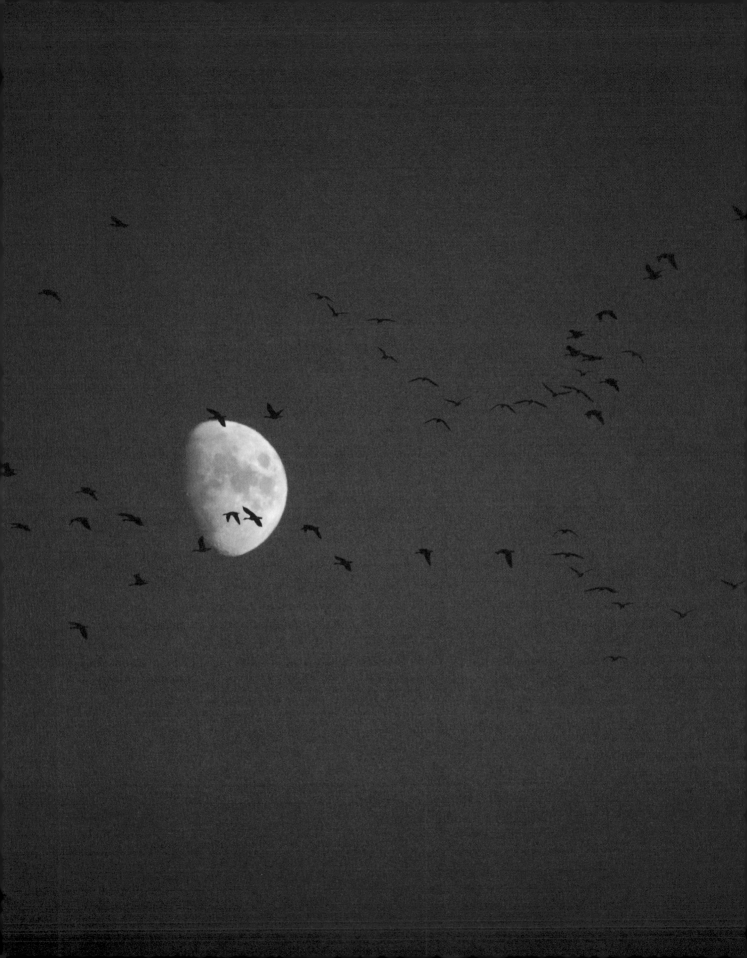

ABOUT THE AUTHORS

Chad Belding, born in Reno, Nevada, is a lifelong sportsman and outdoors enthusiast whose love of the lifestyle was instilled at a very young age by his father, who ensured that Chad and his brothers were encouraged to develop an appreciation of the outdoors at every turn. Chad's passion eventually led him to predator and waterfowl hunting, and he later became involved in competitive duck and goose calling while attending college at The University of Nevada, Reno. Following his graduation with a bachelor's degree, he put his background in business to good use, co-owning and operating several businesses across Nevada, Colorado, and Washington.

In 2008, Chad founded Banded, a video production and merchandising company that specializes in hunting gear and accessories. That same year, he became a part of *The Fowl Life*, which is still airing on The Outdoor Channel. Chad started his podcast *This Life Ain't For Everybody* in 2018, where he covers a wide assortment of themes and topics related to the outdoors. Always looking forward, Chad is also closely involved with The Provider, a new brand that will provide live workshops on dog training, hunting/shooting, and preparing your bounty. When he's not hard at work or spending time with his family, Chad loves music, baseball, and boating and is also a philanthropist working with several charities, including Ronald McDonald House, Freedom Hunters, St. Jude's, and Special Ops Excursions, among others.

Chad Mendes was born and raised in central California, where wrestling, hunting, and fishing were a huge part of his life growing up. He was recruited to wrestle at Cal Poly SLO, where his small-town palate was introduced to a whole new world of cuisines. There he became a two-time NCAA D-I All-American and runner-up during his senior year. After graduating, he moved up to Sacramento and began his UFC career. During his ten years of fighting, he fought for the UFC world title three times, competing against opponents such as Conor McGregor and José Aldo. With hunting being such a huge part of his life still, he teamed up with Chad Belding of *The Fowl Life* to bring readers *The Provider Cookbook*, featuring their favorite recipes.

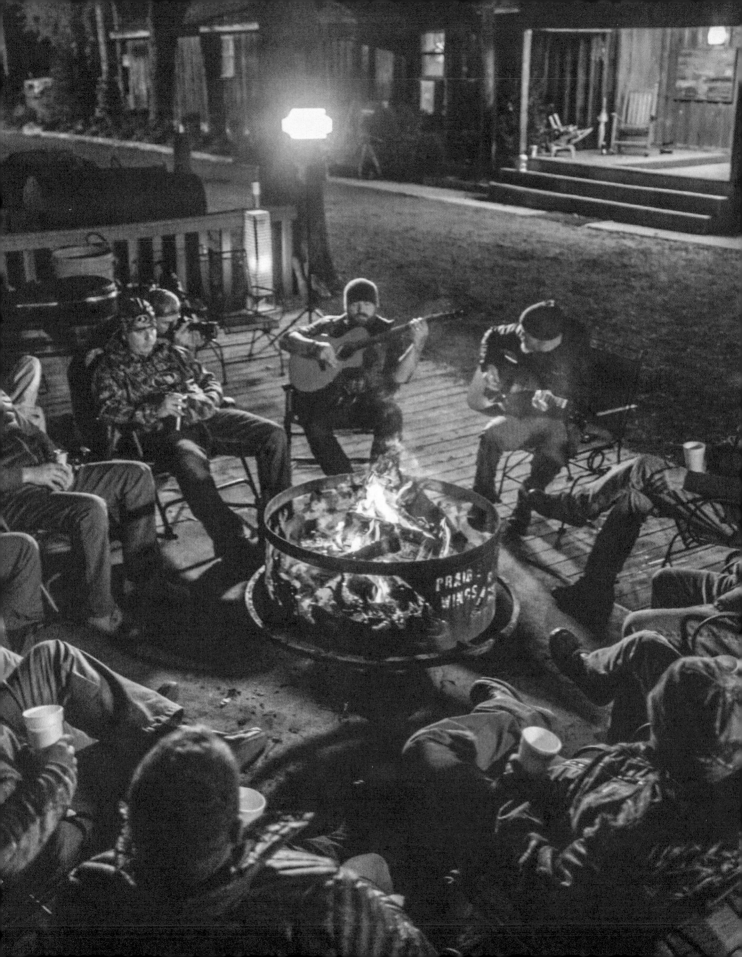